RURAL PEDIATRIC EMERGENCY POCKET GUIDE

DR. MOHAMED ELGENDY, LMCC, CCFP, CANADA

ISBN:

978-1-0697517-1-3 (eBook)
978-1-0697517-0-6 (Paperback)

DISCLAIMER

This pocket guide was developed with the assistance of advanced AI tools to streamline content generation. Every chapter has been thoroughly reviewed, edited, and authenticated by Dr. Mohamed Elgendy, LMCC, CCFP (Canada), ensuring accuracy, credibility, and clinical authenticity. The result is a modern, innovative reference that blends the efficiency of AI with the rigor of professional medical expertise

This booklet summarizes pediatric emergency care principles based on publicly available clinical guidelines and practice statements. It does not reproduce proprietary tables, figures, algorithms, or distinctive wording from subscription-only sources. Content is for education and exam preparation; it is not a substitute for clinical judgment, institutional policies, or local protocols.

Clinical responsibility remains with the treating clinician. Always consult current local guidelines, official product monographs, and institutional pathways. Verify drug doses and contraindications with authoritative sources prior to use.

ABOUT THE AUTHOR

Dr. Mohamed Elgendy is a licensed Canadian physician with the Licentiate of the Medical Council of Canada (LMCC) and Certification in Family Medicine (CCFP) from the College of Family Physicians of Canada. He has several years of hands-on experience as both a rural emergency physician and a family doctor, currently practicing in Saskatchewan, Canada. With a deep commitment to improving healthcare delivery in underserved communities, Dr. Elgendy focuses on practical, evidence-based medicine tailored to the realities of rural practice. His work bridges the gap between academic medicine and frontline care, offering accessible resources to help clinicians make confident, life-saving decisions in resource-limited settings

DEDICATION

This book is dedicated to the children of Rural and remote communities, whose resilience and courage inspire the work we do; to the healthcare providers who face pediatric emergencies with skill, compassion, and determination, often in challenging circumstances; and to my family, whose unwavering support and understanding make this journey possible.

— Dr. Mohamed Elgendy

TABLE OF CONTENTS

CHAPTER 1:
Anaphylaxis & Severe Allergic Reaction

Overview

Anaphylaxis is a severe, life-threatening allergic reaction involving multiple organ systems, often triggered by foods, insect stings, medications, or unknown allergens. It typically develops rapidly and requires immediate recognition and epinephrine administration. Early treatment is crucial to prevent airway compromise and shock.

Red Flags – "Don't Miss" Features

1. Rapid onset (minutes to 2 hours) after allergen exposure
2. Skin/mucosal involvement (urticaria, flushing, angioedema)
3. Respiratory compromise: stridor, wheeze, dyspnea, hypoxia
4. Hypotension, shock, collapse
5. GI symptoms (vomiting, diarrhea, cramping) in combination with above
6. Voice change, throat tightness, or difficulty swallowing

Initial Assessment in the Rural ER

1. ABCs with rapid airway and breathing assessment
2. Oxygen saturation, pulse, BP monitoring
3. Identify possible trigger from history (food, insect, drug, latex)
4. Assess skin, respiratory, cardiovascular, and GI symptoms
5. Time since onset and prior anaphylaxis history
6. Stabilization Protocol
7. **Immediate IM epinephrine** in lateral thigh:
8. 0.01 mg/kg of 1:1000 solution (max 0.3 mg for <30 kg, max 0.5 mg for >30 kg)
9. Repeat q5–15 min if no improvement

Supportive Measures:

1. High-flow O2 via mask
2. IV access and isotonic fluid bolus (20 mL/kg)
3. Position supine with legs elevated (unless respiratory distress worsens)

Adjuncts (after epinephrine):

1. Diphenhydramine 1 mg/kg IV/IM (max 50 mg)
2. Ranitidine 1 mg/kg IV (optional)
3. Methylprednisolone 1–2 mg/kg IV
4. Salbutamol MDI or neb if bronchospasm present

Investigations

1. Diagnosis is clinical—do not delay treatment for investigations
2. Consider glucose, CBC, electrolytes if IV access obtained
3. Tryptase level (if available) for later confirmation (not urgent)
4. ECG and chest x-ray if unstable or persistent symptoms

Differential Diagnosis

1. Anaphylaxis (classic multisystem reaction)
2. Vasovagal syncope
3. Asthma exacerbation
4. Vocal cord dysfunction
5. Sepsis or shock of other origin
6. Panic attack (if mild symptoms)

Management in the Rural Setting

1. Always give IM epinephrine as first-line; delay worsens outcomes
2. Monitor continuously for rebound reaction
3. Educate family on use of epinephrine auto-injector before discharge
4. Prescribe EpiPen Junior or EpiPen based on weight
5. Consider 4–6 hours of observation even if symptoms resolve

Disposition and Transfer Criteria

1. **Observe in rural ER** if stable and improving after epinephrine

Transfer if:

2. Requires >2 doses of epinephrine
3. Hypotension, airway swelling, or respiratory failure
4. No access to appropriate monitoring or pediatric support
5. Discharge with EpiPen and allergist referral if appropriate

Parental Communication & Reassurance

1. Emphasize rapid epinephrine use in future exposures
2. Explain possible biphasic reaction and need for observation
3. Provide education on allergen avoidance and emergency action plan
4. Arrange allergy follow-up or testing if not already known trigger

Documentation Essentials

1. Time of onset, suspected trigger, symptoms
2. Time and dose of epinephrine and other meds
3. Vital signs, clinical course, and disposition
4. Return precautions and EpiPen prescription

Practical Pearls for Rural Docs

1. Epinephrine is first-line—antihistamines and steroids are supportive only
2. IM route preferred over IV unless in extremis
3. Always monitor for biphasic reactions (can occur 4–8 hours later)
4. Always send child home with an epinephrine auto-injector

CHAPTER 2:
Appendicitis – Atypical Presentations

Overview

Appendicitis is a common surgical emergency in children, but atypical presentations can delay diagnosis. Younger children, infants, and those with altered anatomy may present with nonspecific symptoms. Awareness of atypical signs is crucial in rural emergency settings to avoid complications like perforation.

Red Flags – "Don't Miss" Features

1. Abdominal pain that is diffuse or poorly localized
2. Vomiting and anorexia
3. Fever that may be absent or low-grade
4. Diarrhea or urinary symptoms mimicking other conditions
5. Irritability or lethargy in younger children
6. Signs of peritonitis or sepsis in advanced cases

Initial Assessment in the Rural ER

1. Assess ABCs and hydration status
2. Detailed history focusing on onset, location, and character of pain
3. Abdominal exam for tenderness, guarding, rebound, and masses
4. Consider differential diagnoses including UTI, gastroenteritis, constipation
5. Monitor vital signs closely

Stabilization Protocol

1. Provide IV fluids for dehydration
2. Administer analgesia cautiously to avoid masking signs
3. NPO status in preparation for surgery
4. Initiate antibiotics if perforation suspected or planned surgery
5. Monitor for signs of deterioration

Investigations

1. CBC with differential and CRP
2. Urinalysis to rule out UTI
3. Abdominal ultrasound (first line in children)
4. CT abdomen if ultrasound inconclusive and high suspicion
5. Pregnancy test in post-pubertal females

Differential Diagnosis

1. Acute gastroenteritis
2. Urinary tract infection
3. Mesenteric adenitis
4. Constipation
5. Pelvic inflammatory disease or ovarian torsion

Management in the Rural Setting

1. Stabilize and maintain hydration
2. Provide analgesia and monitor clinical progression
3. Arrange urgent transfer for surgical consultation
4. Initiate antibiotics if perforation suspected
5. Communicate closely with receiving center

Disposition and Transfer Criteria

1. Transfer urgently if suspected appendicitis or complications
2. Admit locally only if diagnosis unclear and stable with close observation
3. Provide clear transfer documentation

Parental Communication & Reassurance

1. Explain the need for timely diagnosis and possible surgery
2. Discuss atypical presentations and importance of monitoring
3. Reassure about outcomes with early treatment
4. Provide clear instructions on when to return immediately

Documentation Essentials

1. Detailed pain history and exam findings
2. Vital signs and hydration status
3. Imaging and lab results
4. Communication and transfer details

Practical Pearls for Rural Docs

1. Appendicitis can present atypically especially in young children
2. Early ultrasound can aid diagnosis and reduce radiation exposure
3. Avoid delay in transfer for suspected cases
4. Use analgesia judiciously but do not withhold pain relief

CHAPTER 3:
Asthma Exacerbation (Mild to Life-Threatening)

Overview

Asthma is a chronic inflammatory condition of the airways and a common cause of pediatric emergency visits. Exacerbations range from mild to life-threatening and require prompt assessment, bronchodilator therapy, and supportive care. Rural physicians must quickly recognize severity and initiate treatment while preparing for possible transfer in severe cases.

Red Flags – "Don't Miss" Features

1. Silent chest (minimal air entry despite respiratory effort)
2. Inability to speak or feed
3. Severe accessory muscle use, nasal flaring, retractions
4. Cyanosis, altered mental status
5. O2 saturation <92% on room air
6. Exhaustion or bradycardia (impending respiratory failure)

Initial Assessment in the Rural ER

1. ABCs and oxygen saturation
2. Respiratory rate, effort, auscultation (wheezing vs silent)
3. Assess ability to talk, eat, or drink
4. Classify as mild, moderate, or severe exacerbation
5. Vital signs and brief focused history (onset, triggers, previous ICU admissions)

Stabilization Protocol

Mild to moderate:

1. Salbutamol MDI with spacer: 4–10 puffs q20min x3 doses, then reassess
2. Ipratropium MDI: 4 puffs q20min x3 doses (moderate to severe)
3. Oral dexamethasone 0.6 mg/kg (max 16 mg) or prednisone

Severe to life-threatening:

1. Oxygen to maintain SpO2 ≥94%
2. Nebulized salbutamol 0.15 mg/kg/dose (max 5 mg) q20min
3. Nebulized ipratropium 250 mcg q20min x3
4. IV methylprednisolone 1–2 mg/kg (if unable to take PO)
5. Consider magnesium sulfate IV 25–50 mg/kg over 20 min (max 2 g)
6. Prepare for intubation if deteriorating (consult early)

Investigations

1. Pulse oximetry (continuous)
2. Capillary or venous blood gas (if severe)
3. Chest x-ray only if diagnostic uncertainty or poor response
4. Electrolytes if giving multiple beta-agonist doses (monitor K+)
5. CBC and viral swab not routinely needed

Differential Diagnosis

1. Asthma
2. Bronchiolitis (in <2 years old)
3. Foreign body aspiration
4. Pneumonia
5. Anaphylaxis
6. Vocal cord dysfunction

Management in the Rural Setting

1. Titrate bronchodilators based on severity
2. Give corticosteroids early (PO preferred if not vomiting)
3. Space salbutamol puffs with spacer if possible (preferred over neb if mild)
4. Educate about inhaler technique if child is stable
5. Use weight-based dosing and monitor for toxicity (tachycardia, tremor)

Disposition and Transfer Criteria

1. **Discharge** if mild, improving after 60–90 min, SpO2 >94% on room air, able to eat/drink, and reliable follow-up
2. **Observe** in ER or short stay unit if moderate and improving with treatment

Transfer if:

1. Severe or worsening despite treatment
2. Unable to maintain SpO2 >92%
3. Exhaustion, altered LOC, or silent chest
4. Requires IV meds or potential for intubation

Parental Communication & Reassurance

1. Provide clear instructions on inhaler use and frequency
2. Discuss need for asthma action plan and follow-up
3. Warn about signs of deterioration and when to return
4. Emphasize importance of adherence and environmental triggers

Documentation Essentials

1. Severity classification and vital signs
2. Medication doses, frequency, and response to treatment
3. Parental education and discharge/transfer plan
4. Follow-up arranged or recommended

Practical Pearls for Rural Docs

1. Spacer with MDI is as effective as nebulizer for mild/moderate cases
2. Early steroids reduce relapse and hospitalization
3. Nebulized ipratropium improves outcomes in moderate–severe cases
4. Be prepared for deterioration even after initial improvement

CHAPTER 4:
Baby Syndrome / Non-Accidental Trauma

Overview

Shaken Baby Syndrome (SBS), a form of Abusive Head Trauma (AHT), is a serious manifestation of non-accidental trauma (NAT) in infants and young children. It typically involves violent shaking, leading to intracranial injury, retinal hemorrhages, and other signs of trauma. Early identification is critical, as delayed recognition may result in severe neurologic injury or death.

Red Flags – "Don't Miss" Features

1. Inconsistent or vague history of trauma
2. Delay in seeking medical attention
3. Seizures, altered consciousness, apnea in infants
4. Retinal hemorrhages, bulging fontanelle
5. Bruises in non-mobile infants (especially on torso, ears, neck, or frenulum)
6. Rib fractures, metaphyseal (corner) fractures, or multiple fractures at different stages of healing
7. Unexplained vomiting or lethargy

Initial Assessment in the Rural ER

1. ABCs: prioritize airway and breathing in altered or apneic infants
2. Full head-to-toe physical exam, including neurologic assessment
3. Measure head circumference
4. Check for bruises, burns, swelling, or tenderness over bones
5. Document caregiver's explanation and behavior carefully

Stabilization Protocol

1. Support airway, breathing, and circulation
2. Administer oxygen, IV fluids if hypotensive
3. Manage seizures promptly (e.g., lorazepam 0.1 mg/kg IV)
4. Maintain normoglycemia and normothermia
5. Prepare for urgent neuroimaging if signs of head trauma present

Investigations

1. CBC, coagulation studies (to rule out bleeding disorders)
2. Head CT (non-contrast) for suspected intracranial injury
3. Skeletal survey (if available) or request at tertiary center
4. Retinal exam by ophthalmology (if available)
5. Toxicology screen if ingestion suspected

Differential Diagnosis

1. Accidental trauma (less likely in non-mobile child)
2. Sepsis/meningitis (can present with altered LOC)
3. Bleeding disorder (e.g., hemophilia)
4. Metabolic disorders (e.g., glutaric aciduria type I)
5. Gastroenteritis or reflux (if vomiting only)

Management in the Rural Setting

1. Stabilize vitals and initiate seizure control
2. Avoid discharge or reassurance without full investigation
3. Ensure proper documentation of findings and caregiver explanations
4. Report immediately to child protection services and document notification
5. Consult pediatric specialists (neurology, ICU, social work)

Disposition and Transfer Criteria

1. **Urgent transfer** to a pediatric trauma or ICU center if:
2. Altered LOC, seizures, suspected intracranial injury
3. Need for neuroimaging, ophthalmology, skeletal survey
4. Always transfer after initial stabilization, even if stable
5. Coordinate with pediatric emergency, PICU, and child protection services

Parental Communication & Reassurance

1. Approach discussion carefully and avoid accusations
2. Explain that certain findings require specialized evaluation
3. Maintain professionalism even if abuse is suspected
4. Ensure child is not discharged to potentially unsafe environment

Documentation Essentials

1. Exact history provided by caregiver (use quotations)
2. Detailed physical exam: bruises, head circumference, neuro status
3. Interventions and response
4. Communication with child protection and transfer center

Practical Pearls for Rural Docs

1. Any injury in a non-mobile infant is suspicious until proven otherwise
2. Retinal hemorrhages + subdural hematomas = highly suggestive of SBS
3. Rib and metaphyseal fractures are classic for abuse
4. Trust your clinical suspicion—mandatory reporting is required in Canada

CHAPTER 5:
Bronchiolitis

Overview

Bronchiolitis is a common lower respiratory tract infection in infants, usually caused by respiratory syncytial virus (RSV). It presents with cough, wheeze, and respiratory distress. Most cases are mild and self-limited, but infants under 6 months and those with comorbidities may develop severe symptoms requiring oxygen, hydration, or transfer.

Red Flags – "Don't Miss" Features

1. Age <3 months or former preterm infant
2. Respiratory rate >70/min or severe retractions
3. Apnea (especially in very young infants)
4. Poor feeding, dehydration
5. O2 saturation <90% on room air
6. Cyanosis, lethargy, or altered mental status

Initial Assessment in the Rural ER

1. Vital signs including oxygen saturation
2. General appearance, work of breathing (grunting, nasal flaring, retractions)
3. Auscultation: wheezes, crackles, decreased breath sounds
4. Feeding history and urine output (hydration)
5. Consider RSV season and exposure history

Stabilization Protocol

1. Ensure airway patency; position upright or prone on parent's chest

2. Administer oxygen via nasal cannula to maintain SpO2 >90–92%
3. Suction nares if copious secretions are present
4. Monitor for apnea and fatigue
5. IV fluids if unable to maintain oral intake

Investigations

1. Diagnosis is clinical; no labs or imaging routinely needed
2. Consider CXR only if atypical features (e.g., high fever, focal findings)
3. RSV/viral testing may help with cohorting but not routine in rural setting
4. Blood glucose if not feeding or irritable

Differential Diagnosis

1. Bronchiolitis (RSV, other viruses)
2. Asthma (rare <1 year, consider in older infants)
3. Pneumonia (especially with focal signs or fever)
4. Foreign body aspiration
5. Sepsis (in neonates)
6. Congenital heart disease

Management in the Rural Setting

1. Supportive care only; no routine use of bronchodilators, steroids, or antibiotics
2. Trial of salbutamol if history of atopy or previous wheeze, but discontinue if no response
3. Nasal suction before feeds
4. Monitor for signs of fatigue, dehydration, or apnea
5. Maintain hydration: oral or IV if needed

Disposition and Transfer Criteria

1. **Discharge** if mild symptoms, feeding well, SpO2 >92%, stable exam
2. **Observe** in ED for feeding or oxygen trial if uncertain

Transfer if:

1. SpO2 <90% on oxygen
2. Moderate-severe distress or apnea
3. Poor oral intake, dehydration
4. Infant <6 weeks or with comorbidities (CHD, chronic lung disease, immunocompromised)

Parental Communication & Reassurance

1. Explain natural course: typically 5–7 days, worst on days 3–4
2. Emphasize nasal suction, hydration, and feeding as key
3. Reassure that antibiotics and puffers usually don't help
4. Discuss when to return (increased work of breathing, poor feeding, less wet diapers)

Documentation Essentials

1. Respiratory rate, oxygen saturation, feeding and hydration status
2. Description of physical findings (e.g., wheeze, retractions)
3. Any trialed interventions (e.g., salbutamol)
4. Disposition decision and parental education

Practical Pearls for Rural Docs

1. Bronchiolitis is viral – avoid unnecessary antibiotics or steroids
2. Infants may tire quickly – observe closely if RR >70 or not feeding
3. Apnea may be the first sign in very young infants
4. Nasal suction can significantly improve feeding and breathing

CHAPTER 6:
Bronchitis

Overview

Bronchitis is inflammation of the bronchi, usually viral in children, presenting with cough, wheezing, and sometimes fever. It is often self-limited and managed supportively. Distinguishing bronchitis from more severe lower respiratory infections is important.

Red Flags – "Don't Miss" Features

1. Persistent or worsening cough beyond 2 weeks
2. High fever or toxic appearance
3. Signs of respiratory distress or hypoxia
4. Hemoptysis or chest pain
5. Underlying chronic lung disease

Initial Assessment in the Rural ER

1. Assess airway, breathing, circulation
2. Vital signs including SpO2 and respiratory rate
3. Auscultation: wheezes, crackles, decreased breath sounds
4. History of cough duration, sputum, exposures, and prior illnesses

Stabilization Protocol

1. Supportive care with hydration and antipyretics
2. Oxygen if hypoxic (SpO2 <92%)
3. Bronchodilators trial if wheezing and suspected reactive airway disease
4. Avoid antibiotics unless bacterial superinfection suspected

Investigations

1. Usually clinical diagnosis; labs and imaging not routinely needed
2. Chest x-ray if suspicion for pneumonia or complications
3. Viral testing if available and affects management

Differential Diagnosis

1. Viral bronchitis
2. Bronchiolitis (younger infants)
3. Pneumonia
4. Asthma exacerbation
5. Foreign body aspiration

Management in the Rural Setting

1. Provide supportive care and monitor for worsening symptoms
2. Educate caregivers on cough management and when to seek care
3. Arrange follow-up if cough persists or worsens

Disposition and Transfer Criteria

1. Discharge if well-appearing, stable vitals, no distress
2. Transfer if respiratory distress, hypoxia, or concern for pneumonia

Parental Communication & Reassurance

1. Explain usual viral nature and expected duration
2. Teach supportive measures like hydration and humidification

3. Warn about signs of worsening or secondary bacterial infection

Documentation Essentials

1. Description of cough and respiratory exam
2. Vital signs and oxygen saturation
3. Treatments given and follow-up instructions

Practical Pearls for Rural Docs

1. Most bronchitis is viral and self-limited
2. Avoid unnecessary antibiotics
3. Distinguish bronchitis from pneumonia by exam and response
4. Persistent cough warrants further evaluation

CHAPTER 7:
COVID-19 & MIS-C

Overview

COVID-19 in children often presents with mild symptoms but can occasionally cause severe respiratory illness. Multisystem Inflammatory Syndrome in Children (MIS-C) is a rare but serious post-infectious complication characterized by systemic inflammation, fever, and multi-organ involvement, occurring weeks after initial infection.

Red Flags – "Don't Miss" Features

1. Persistent fever >38.5°C for >24 hours
2. Hypotension or shock signs
3. Respiratory distress or hypoxia
4. Abdominal pain, vomiting, diarrhea
5. Rash, conjunctivitis, mucous membrane changes
6. Altered mental status or lethargy
7. Elevated inflammatory markers (if labs done)

Initial Assessment in the Rural ER

1. Assess airway, breathing, and circulation
2. Vital signs including oxygen saturation and temperature
3. History of recent COVID-19 infection or exposure
4. Complete physical exam including mucocutaneous findings and abdominal tenderness
5. Evaluate for signs of shock or organ dysfunction

Stabilization Protocol

1. Oxygen to maintain SpO2 >94%
2. IV access and isotonic fluid boluses for shock
3. Supportive care for respiratory distress

4. Empiric antibiotics if bacterial co-infection suspected
5. Early initiation of immunomodulatory therapy (IVIG, steroids) per specialist advice if MIS-C suspected

Investigations

1. CBC, CRP, ESR, ferritin, D-dimer, troponin, BNP
2. SARS-CoV-2 PCR or antigen test
3. Blood cultures and urine analysis
4. Chest X-ray and echocardiogram (if available)
5. ECG and cardiac enzymes for myocarditis

Differential Diagnosis

1. COVID-19 infection (mild to severe)
2. MIS-C (Kawasaki-like syndrome)
3. Sepsis or toxic shock syndrome
4. Viral gastroenteritis
5. Other causes of fever and rash

Management in the Rural Setting

1. Support airway, breathing, and circulation aggressively
2. Monitor for progression to shock or cardiac involvement
3. Provide fluids cautiously to avoid overload
4. Initiate early transfer planning for suspected MIS-C or severe COVID-19
5. Consult infectious disease and pediatric ICU teams promptly

Disposition and Transfer Criteria

Transfer urgently if:

1. Signs of shock, respiratory failure, or altered mental status
2. Suspected MIS-C requiring immunomodulatory treatment
3. Need for advanced cardiac monitoring or critical care
4. Stable patients with mild disease may be managed with close outpatient follow-up

Parental Communication & Reassurance

1. Explain that most children have mild illness but vigilance is necessary
2. Educate about signs of worsening including shock and respiratory distress
3. Discuss infection control measures and isolation
4. Provide clear instructions on when to return to hospital

Documentation Essentials

1. Document history of COVID-19 exposure or infection
2. Vital signs and physical exam findings
3. Labs and imaging results
4. Treatments given and consultation notes
5. Communication with family and transfer details

Practical Pearls for Rural Docs

1. MIS-C may present weeks after mild or asymptomatic COVID-19
2. Cardiac involvement is common and can be severe in MIS-C
3. Early recognition and transfer are key to outcomes

4. Use PPE and follow local infection control protocols

CHAPTER 8:
Cardiac Arrest (PALS Approach)

Overview

Cardiac arrest in children is most often secondary to respiratory failure or shock, unlike adults where it is typically cardiac in origin. Immediate, high-quality CPR and adherence to Pediatric Advanced Life Support (PALS) guidelines dramatically improve survival and neurological outcomes. Early recognition, effective ventilation, and appropriate drug use are critical.

Red Flags – "Don't Miss" Features

1. Unresponsive, no breathing, and no palpable pulse ≥10 seconds
2. Agonal breathing or gasping only
3. Bradycardia with poor perfusion (pre-arrest warning)
4. Hypoxia, apnea, or signs of severe shock leading to arrest

Initial Assessment in the Rural ER

1. Check responsiveness, airway, breathing, and circulation
2. Activate emergency response/code blue system
3. Begin CPR immediately if no pulse or <60 bpm with signs of poor perfusion
4. Use Broselow tape for weight-based dosing and equipment sizing
5. Place monitoring: cardiac leads, SpO2, and ETCO2 (if intubated)

Stabilization Protocol

1. **CPR Guidelines (PALS 2020):**
2. **Rate**: 100–120 compressions/min
3. **Depth**: At least 1/3 AP diameter (4 cm in infants, 5 cm in children)
4. **Ratio**: 15:2 (2-rescuer) or 30:2 (single-rescuer)
5. **Allow full chest recoil and minimize interruptions**
6. Rotate compressors every 2 minutes

Airway & Breathing:

1. Bag-mask ventilation initially; intubate if prolonged or ineffective BVM
2. Ventilation rate: 1 breath every 2–3 sec (20–30 breaths/min) if intubated

Defibrillation:

1. Use AED or manual defibrillator ASAP in VF/pulseless VT
2. First shock: 2 J/kg → Second and subsequent shocks: 4 J/kg (max 10 J/kg or adult dose)

Medications:

1. Epinephrine 0.01 mg/kg IV/IO (1:10,000) q3–5 min during arrest
2. Amiodarone 5 mg/kg IV/IO bolus for shock-refractory VF/pVT (may repeat x2)
3. Lidocaine (alternative): 1 mg/kg IV/IO loading dose

Investigations

1. Glucose (POC) – treat hypoglycemia
2. Blood gas, electrolytes, calcium, magnesium if prolonged arrest
3. ECG after ROSC or during arrhythmia

4. Consider reversible causes (4 Hs & 4 Ts)

Differential Diagnosis (4 Hs & 4 Ts)

1. **Hypoxia**
2. **Hypovolemia**
3. **Hypo-/Hyperkalemia**,**Hypoglycemia**, **Hypothermia**
4. **Tension pneumothorax**
5. **Tamponade (cardiac)**
6. **Toxins/Drugs**
7. **Thromboembolism (rare in peds)**

Management in the Rural Setting

1. Focus on high-quality CPR and early epinephrine
2. Defibrillate if indicated
3. Secure IV/IO access; use intraosseous if IV fails
4. Continue CPR and drug cycles until ROSC or decision to stop
5. Prepare for transfer after ROSC (optimize ventilation, fluids, vasopressors)

Disposition and Transfer Criteria

1. **After ROSC (Return of Spontaneous Circulation):**
2. Stabilize airway, breathing, circulation
3. Maintain normoxia, normocapnia, and normothermia
4. Arrange urgent PICU transfer with continuous monitoring
5. **If no ROSC after 20–30 min and no reversible cause found**: consider cessation per guidelines and after discussion with family and team

Parental Communication & Reassurance

1. Assign a team member to update and support the family
2. Be honest and compassionate about the condition and interventions
3. Involve them in decision-making as appropriate
4. Provide written summary and arrange grief support if outcome is poor

Documentation Essentials

1. Time of arrest, CPR initiation, ROSC (if achieved)
2. Airway method, rhythm changes, shocks given
3. All medication doses and times
4. Communication with family and transport coordination

Practical Pearls for Rural Docs

1. Most pediatric arrests are respiratory → oxygenation is critical
2. Use Broselow tape to guide resuscitation meds and equipment
3. Defibrillate early in VF/pVT and administer epinephrine without delay
4. Always debrief team after a pediatric code—emotional and educational

CHAPTER 9:
Constipation – Red Flags & Initial Management

Overview

Constipation is a common pediatric complaint that can cause significant discomfort and parental concern. While often functional, certain cases may suggest underlying pathology requiring urgent intervention. In rural settings, careful evaluation is essential to rule out red flags and initiate appropriate treatment.

Red Flags – "Don't Miss" Features

1. Delayed passage of meconium >48 hours after birth (Hirschsprung's suspicion)
2. Vomiting (especially bilious) or abdominal distension
3. Weight loss or failure to thrive
4. Anal fissures with bleeding or severe pain
5. Neurogenic signs (e.g., abnormal lower limb tone or reflexes)
6. Spinal anomalies or sacral dimples
7. Recent onset with severe pain or complete obstruction

Initial Assessment in the Rural ER

1. Assess hydration status and abdominal exam (distension, tenderness, masses)
2. Review diet, fluid intake, and stooling pattern
3. Check for signs of systemic illness or developmental delay
4. Inspect perianal area for fissures or signs of Hirschsprung's disease
5. Assess for spinal abnormalities and neurological findings

Stabilization Protocol

1. Treat pain and anxiety with age-appropriate analgesia
2. Gentle rectal stimulation or glycerin suppository in infants if indicated
3. Consider disimpaction if fecal mass is palpable (oral PEG or rectal enema)
4. Avoid repeated enemas in neonates or undifferentiated cases without specialist input
5. Start oral rehydration if dehydrated

Investigations

1. No tests needed for typical functional constipation
2. Abdominal X-ray only if diagnosis unclear or severe distension
3. Consider TSH, calcium, and celiac screen in chronic cases with red flags
4. Barium enema or anorectal manometry if Hirschsprung's suspected (refer out)

Differential Diagnosis

1. Functional constipation (most common)
2. Hirschsprung's disease
3. Spinal dysraphism
4. Cystic fibrosis
5. Anorectal malformations
6. Hypothyroidism

Management in the Rural Setting

1. Education about high-fiber diet and fluid intake
2. Initiate oral polyethylene glycol (PEG 3350) for disimpaction if needed
3. Introduce maintenance therapy after disimpaction

4. Reassure families that functional constipation is common and treatable
5. Avoid rectal exams in neonates unless guided by a specialist

Disposition and Transfer Criteria

1. Transfer if signs of obstruction, failure to thrive, or neurological concerns
2. Refer infants with delayed meconium or suspected Hirschsprung's
3. Follow-up in outpatient care if mild and improving on therapy

Parental Communication & Reassurance

1. Explain that most cases are functional and improve with routine changes
2. Provide written instructions for PEG use and dietary modifications
3. Review red flags and when to return (e.g., vomiting, distension, no improvement)

Documentation Essentials

1. Detailed history of stooling patterns, diet, and red flags
2. Physical exam including abdominal and neurological findings
3. Treatment administered in ER and response
4. Disposition plan and follow-up advice

Practical Pearls for Rural Docs

1. Functional constipation is a diagnosis of exclusion
2. Do not delay referral for infants with delayed meconium or significant red flags
3. Oral PEG is safe, effective, and better tolerated than enemas in children
4. Early dietary advice can prevent recurrence

CHAPTER 10:
Croup (Laryngotracheitis)

Overview

Croup (viral laryngotracheitis) is a common respiratory illness in children aged 6 months to 6 years, caused primarily by parainfluenza virus. It presents with a barking cough, hoarseness, and inspiratory stridor due to upper airway inflammation. Most cases are mild, but severe cases can lead to airway obstruction and require emergent treatment and possible transfer.

Red Flags – "Don't Miss" Features

1. Stridor at rest
2. Retractions, nasal flaring, or tracheal tugging
3. Drooling or inability to swallow (consider epiglottitis)
4. Cyanosis or altered LOC
5. Poor air entry or silent chest
6. Lack of response to initial treatment

Initial Assessment in the Rural ER

1. Avoid agitating the child; observe calmly from a distance
2. Assess for stridor (at rest vs exertion), work of breathing, oxygen saturation
3. Vital signs (RR, HR, temp), mental status
4. Look for signs of impending airway compromise (lethargy, cyanosis)
5. Evaluate for differential diagnoses (e.g., epiglottitis, foreign body)

Stabilization Protocol

1. **Mild croup** (no stridor at rest, mild retractions):
2. Oral dexamethasone 0.6 mg/kg (max 10 mg)
3. **Moderate to severe croup** (stridor at rest, retractions, distress):
4. Nebulized epinephrine 5 mL of 1:1000 solution via nebulizer
5. Dexamethasone 0.6 mg/kg PO/IM/IV (max 10 mg)
6. Monitor closely for rebound symptoms (within 2–3 hours)
7. Keep child calm, upright; avoid unnecessary interventions

Investigations

1. Diagnosis is clinical; no labs or imaging usually required
2. Avoid throat exam if suspecting epiglottitis
3. Neck x-ray ("steeple sign") rarely needed and should not delay treatment
4. Consider CXR only if atypical presentation or poor response to treatment

Differential Diagnosis

1. Croup (viral laryngotracheitis)
2. Epiglottitis (drooling, toxic, rapid onset)
3. Foreign body aspiration
4. Bacterial tracheitis
5. Retropharyngeal abscess
6. Anaphylaxis (if sudden onset with stridor and swelling)

Management in the Rural Setting

1. Administer dexamethasone early in all suspected cases
2. Nebulized epinephrine for moderate–severe cases or if stridor at rest
3. Keep child with parent to minimize distress

4. Observe for 2–3 hours after nebulized epinephrine to assess for rebound
5. Prepare for airway support if deterioration occurs

Disposition and Transfer Criteria

1. **Discharge** if mild symptoms, no stridor at rest, good response to dexamethasone
2. **Observe in ER** if received nebulized epinephrine (for at least 2 hours)

Transfer if:

1. Stridor persists at rest or requires multiple epi treatments
2. Increased work of breathing or altered LOC
3. Need for airway support or intensive monitoring

Parental Communication & Reassurance

1. Explain that croup is usually viral and self-limited
2. Teach signs of worsening: stridor at rest, breathing difficulty, cyanosis
3. Encourage hydration and use of cool mist/humidified air at home
4. Provide return precautions and dosing info for steroids if needed

Documentation Essentials

1. Description of symptoms and severity (Westley Croup Score optional)
2. Medications given (dexamethasone, epinephrine) and response
3. Observation period and re-evaluation findings
4. Parental instructions and discharge/transfer details

Practical Pearls for Rural Docs

1. Early dexamethasone reduces hospitalization and relapse
2. Nebulized epinephrine has rapid onset but short duration—observe after use
3. Avoid agitating the child—no IVs or exams unless absolutely necessary
4. If deterioration: prepare for airway management and transfer

CHAPTER 11:
Dehydration with Hypovolemic Shock

Overview

Hypovolemic shock in children is most commonly due to severe dehydration, typically from gastroenteritis, with fluid losses through vomiting, diarrhea, or both. Infants and young children are especially vulnerable due to limited fluid reserves. Early recognition and aggressive fluid resuscitation are life-saving.

Red Flags – "Don't Miss" Features

1. Lethargy or altered mental status
2. Tachycardia (early sign), bradycardia (late/ominous)
3. Delayed capillary refill (>3 seconds)
4. Cool, mottled extremities
5. Minimal or absent urine output
6. Hypotension (late and pre-arrest sign in children)
7. Sunken eyes, sunken fontanelle, absent tears

Initial Assessment in the Rural ER

1. ABCs and rapid vital signs
2. Weight, recent fluid losses, feeding history, urine output
3. Physical exam: mucous membranes, skin turgor, pulses, mental status
4. Assess level of dehydration (mild, moderate, severe)
5. Consider possible causes: infection, DKA, hemorrhage

Stabilization Protocol

1. **Establish IV or IO access immediately**
2. **Fluid resuscitation with isotonic fluids (NS or RL):**
3. 20 mL/kg bolus over 10–20 minutes

4. Repeat as needed up to 60 mL/kg while monitoring response
5. Monitor HR, perfusion, LOC between boluses
6. Oxygen via face mask to support tissue perfusion
7. Consider antibiotics if sepsis cannot be ruled out
8. Check blood glucose and treat hypoglycemia if present

Investigations

1. Point-of-care glucose
2. Electrolytes, BUN, creatinine
3. CBC, lactate if sepsis suspected
4. Venous blood gas (acidosis)
5. Urinalysis (dehydration or underlying infection)

Differential Diagnosis

1. Gastroenteritis-related dehydration (most common)
2. Sepsis (may overlap clinically)
3. Diabetic ketoacidosis
4. Hemorrhage or trauma
5. Adrenal crisis (rare)
6. Intussusception or surgical abdomen

Management in the Rural Setting

1. Aggressive volume resuscitation is key—do not delay for labs
2. Reassess after each bolus: HR, perfusion, LOC, urine output
3. If improving, begin maintenance and replacement fluids
4. Monitor electrolytes and glucose closely
5. Prepare for transfer if not stabilizing after 60 mL/kg or if deteriorating

Disposition and Transfer Criteria

1. **Admit locally** if improved with fluids and stable for oral intake

Transfer urgently if:

1. Persistent shock after 60 mL/kg fluid boluses
2. Altered LOC or hemodynamic instability
3. Need for ICU-level monitoring or IV infusion pumps
4. Severe electrolyte disturbances or unclear diagnosis

Parental Communication & Reassurance

1. Explain severity and need for urgent fluid replacement
2. Educate on signs of dehydration and oral rehydration at home
3. Reinforce safe feeding practices during illness
4. Provide discharge instructions if improving and sent home

Documentation Essentials

1. Degree of dehydration and clinical signs on presentation
2. All fluid boluses (amount, type, time)
3. Response to fluids: HR, BP, perfusion, mental status
4. Parental discussion, disposition plan, follow-up

Practical Pearls for Rural Docs

1. Hypotension is a late sign in pediatric shock—act early based on perfusion
2. IO access is fast and effective if IV fails
3. Avoid dextrose-containing boluses unless hypoglycemic
4. Use Broselow tape for weight-based dosing if unsure of exact weight

CHAPTER 12:
Diabetic Ketoacidosis (DKA)

Overview

Diabetic ketoacidosis (DKA) is a life-threatening complication of type 1 diabetes characterized by hyperglycemia, ketosis, and metabolic acidosis. Early recognition and management are essential to prevent cerebral edema and other complications, especially in rural settings where pediatric endocrinology support may be limited.

Red Flags – "Don't Miss" Features

1. Polyuria, polydipsia, weight loss
2. Vomiting, abdominal pain
3. Kussmaul respirations (deep, rapid breathing)
4. Altered mental status or lethargy
5. Dehydration signs: dry mucous membranes, tachycardia
6. Fruity (acetone) breath odor

Initial Assessment in the Rural ER

1. Assess airway, breathing, and circulation
2. Obtain vital signs and mental status evaluation
3. Measure blood glucose and ketones if point-of-care testing available
4. Evaluate hydration and neurological status
5. Obtain history of diabetes diagnosis and insulin adherence

Stabilization Protocol

1. Establish IV access and begin fluid resuscitation with isotonic saline
2. Correct electrolyte imbalances, especially potassium
3. Initiate insulin therapy after fluid resuscitation started

4. Monitor glucose, ketones, electrolytes, and mental status closely
5. Prepare for transfer to pediatric ICU if indicated

Investigations

1. Blood glucose, serum ketones or urine ketones
2. Serum electrolytes, blood gas (pH, bicarbonate)
3. CBC, blood cultures if infection suspected
4. Serum osmolality and renal function tests

Differential Diagnosis

1. DKA due to new-onset or poorly controlled diabetes
2. Hyperglycemic hyperosmolar state (rare in children)
3. Gastroenteritis causing dehydration
4. Sepsis or other causes of metabolic acidosis

Management in the Rural Setting

1. Correct dehydration cautiously to avoid cerebral edema
2. Replace potassium unless hyperkalemia present
3. Administer insulin infusion with careful monitoring
4. Avoid rapid glucose lowering
5. Provide supportive care and treat underlying triggers

Disposition and Transfer Criteria

1. Transfer to pediatric ICU for:
2. Altered mental status or coma
3. Severe electrolyte abnormalities
4. Inability to manage fluids or insulin locally
5. Stable mild cases may be managed with close monitoring and endocrinology input

Parental Communication & Reassurance

1. Explain the emergency nature and treatment plan
2. Educate about diabetes management and preventing DKA
3. Reassure about prognosis with prompt care
4. Discuss signs of worsening and when to seek help

Documentation Essentials

1. Blood glucose and ketone levels
2. Vital signs and neurological assessment
3. Fluid and insulin administration details
4. Communication with family and transfer notes

Practical Pearls for Rural Docs

1. Avoid fluid overload and rapid glucose drops to prevent cerebral edema
2. Potassium replacement is critical but must be carefully monitored
3. Early transfer and multidisciplinary care improve outcomes
4. Educate families on sick day management and insulin adherence

CHAPTER 13:
Dog Bites & Wound Infections

Overview

Dog bites are a frequent pediatric emergency, particularly in rural communities. While many are minor, they can lead to significant complications such as soft tissue infection, tendon or bone involvement, and rarely rabies. Proper wound cleaning, early antibiotic treatment, and vaccination updates are critical.

Red Flags – "Don't Miss" Features

1. Deep puncture wounds, crush injuries, or avulsions
2. Bites involving the face, scalp, hands, feet, or genitals
3. Signs of local infection (erythema, warmth, swelling, pus)
4. Systemic signs: fever, lethargy, or sepsis
5. Wounds with suspected joint, bone, or tendon involvement
6. Unvaccinated or stray dog bites (risk of rabies)
7. Delayed presentation >12–24 hours after injury

Initial Assessment in the Rural ER

1. Stabilize ABCs if needed; assess pain and bleeding
2. Gather history: dog ownership, vaccination status, provoked vs unprovoked attack
3. Examine wound size, location, depth, and signs of infection
4. Assess neurovascular status distal to the bite
5. Check tetanus and rabies immunization history

Stabilization Protocol

1. Irrigate wound with copious normal saline or soapy water for 10–15 minutes
2. Debride devitalized or contaminated tissue

3. Apply sterile dressing after cleaning
4. Control bleeding with direct pressure
5. Administer tetanus booster if indicated
6. Start empiric antibiotics (e.g., amoxicillin-clavulanate)
7. Consider rabies post-exposure prophylaxis (HRIG + vaccine) if criteria met

Investigations

1. Usually clinical diagnosis based on wound
2. Wound culture if purulence or delayed presentation
3. X-ray for suspected fractures, retained teeth, or foreign bodies
4. CBC, CRP if signs of systemic infection

Differential Diagnosis

1. Uncomplicated dog bite (no infection or deep involvement)
2. Infected bite wound – cellulitis or abscess
3. Tenosynovitis, septic arthritis, or osteomyelitis
4. Rabies exposure (rare but fatal)
5. Tetanus (if unimmunized)

Management in the Rural Setting

1. Thorough wound cleaning and debridement
2. Start oral antibiotics in high-risk or moderate/severe wounds
3. Avoid primary closure unless wound is facial or clean and <6 hrs old
4. Administer tetanus booster as per guidelines
5. Rabies PEP if high-risk: start in ER and refer to public health
6. Discharge with wound care instructions and follow-up within 48 hrs

Disposition and Transfer Criteria

1. Transfer for surgical repair of large/deep facial wounds
2. Refer to tertiary center for suspected bone or joint involvement
3. Urgent transfer if systemic infection or suspected rabies exposure and vaccine/HRIG not available

Parental Communication & Reassurance

1. Most bites heal well with proper care and antibiotics
2. Explain importance of wound care and completing antibiotic course
3. Advise on signs of infection and when to return to hospital
4. Reinforce need for vaccination updates (tetanus, rabies)

Documentation Essentials

1. Time, mechanism, and setting of injury
2. Dog description and rabies vaccination status (if known)
3. Wound location, depth, signs of infection
4. Neurovascular exam findings
5. Treatments administered: irrigation, antibiotics, tetanus, rabies PEP
6. Instructions given and follow-up arrangements

Practical Pearls for Rural Docs

1. Clean early and thoroughly — this prevents most complications
2. Do not primarily close puncture wounds unless on the face
3. Start antibiotics early in high-risk wounds
4. Consult public health for any rabies PEP questions or shortages
5. Facial wounds should be repaired by specialists if deep or extensive

CHAPTER 14:
Epiglottitis

Overview

Epiglottitis is a rapidly progressive and potentially fatal infection of the epiglottis, usually caused by Haemophilus influenzae type B (Hib) in unvaccinated children. It causes severe upper airway obstruction and must be recognized early. Prompt airway management and antibiotic therapy are lifesaving.

Red Flags – "Don't Miss" Features

1. Sudden onset high fever, sore throat, and drooling
2. Tripod position (sitting forward with neck extended)
3. Muffled or "hot potato" voice
4. Stridor (usually late sign)
5. Difficulty swallowing or speaking
6. Cyanosis or altered mental status

Initial Assessment in the Rural ER

1. **Do NOT attempt to visualize the throat or use tongue depressor**
2. Minimize agitation; allow child to stay in position of comfort (often tripod)
3. Observe from a distance: look for drooling, stridor, labored breathing
4. Monitor vital signs and oxygen saturation continuously
5. Prepare for immediate airway intervention

Stabilization Protocol

1. **Do not separate child from caregiver or force interventions**
2. Administer humidified oxygen if tolerated

3. Keep resuscitation and airway equipment ready: bag-valve mask, suction, intubation tools, cricothyrotomy kit
4. Arrange for urgent intubation in controlled environment (preferably OR or with anesthesia support)
5. Administer IV antibiotics after airway secured:
6. Ceftriaxone 100 mg/kg/day IV or Cefotaxime 200 mg/kg/day IV
7. Consider vancomycin if MRSA suspected

Investigations

1. Diagnosis is clinical—do NOT delay airway management for tests
2. Lateral neck x-ray (if safe to obtain) may show "thumbprint sign"
3. Blood cultures after securing airway
4. Avoid bloodwork or imaging if child is unstable or agitated

Differential Diagnosis

1. Epiglottitis (true emergency)
2. Croup (slower onset, barking cough, no drooling)
3. Retropharyngeal abscess
4. Foreign body aspiration
5. Anaphylaxis (if associated with urticaria or hypotension)
6. Peritonsillar abscess (usually older children, less airway risk)

Management in the Rural Setting

1. Prioritize calm environment and airway protection
2. Avoid unnecessary IVs or exams until airway secured
3. Start broad-spectrum IV antibiotics only after airway is managed
4. Consult pediatric ENT/anesthesia/ICU team early if available
5. Prepare for transport if definitive airway not available locally

Disposition and Transfer Criteria

1. **All cases require urgent transfer** to a pediatric ICU or tertiary care center
2. If airway secured: transfer stable with monitoring
3. If airway not secured: urgent air or ground transport with pre-alert to receiving team
4. Transport must include personnel skilled in pediatric airway management

Parental Communication & Reassurance

1. Explain the seriousness of the condition and need for emergency airway support
2. Allow caregiver to remain with child during initial stabilization
3. Reassure that early intervention can be lifesaving
4. Avoid panic or alarming the child/parent unnecessarily

Documentation Essentials

1. Onset and progression of symptoms (fever, drooling, stridor)
2. Positioning and appearance on exam (e.g., tripod, muffled voice)
3. Medications and airway interventions attempted or planned
4. Time and content of calls to consultants and transfer teams

Practical Pearls for Rural Docs

1. Never attempt to examine the throat in suspected epiglottitis
2. Stridor is a late and ominous sign—act on earlier signs like drooling and tripod position
3. Avoid delays—airway intervention and antibiotics save lives
4. Think epiglottitis in any toxic-appearing child with drooling and no cough

CHAPTER 15:
Failure to Thrive – Acute Evaluation

Overview

Failure to thrive (FTT) refers to inadequate growth or weight gain in infants and children. Acute evaluation focuses on identifying underlying causes such as nutritional deficiencies, chronic illnesses, or psychosocial factors. Early diagnosis and intervention improve outcomes, especially in rural settings where resources may be limited.

Red Flags – "Don't Miss" Features

1. Severe malnutrition signs (muscle wasting, edema)
2. Developmental delays
3. Persistent vomiting or diarrhea
4. Signs of chronic illness (heart murmurs, respiratory distress)
5. Poor feeding behavior or neglect
6. Weight or height below 3rd percentile or crossing growth percentiles downward

Initial Assessment in the Rural ER

1. Measure weight, height, and head circumference accurately
2. Obtain detailed dietary and feeding history
3. Assess developmental milestones and behavior
4. Perform full physical exam focusing on signs of systemic disease
5. Review social history including family dynamics and access to food

Stabilization Protocol

1. Address immediate concerns such as dehydration or infections
2. Begin nutritional support with guidance from dietitians if available
3. Treat underlying medical conditions promptly
4. Monitor vitals and hydration status
5. Plan for close follow-up and support services

Investigations

1. CBC, electrolytes, blood glucose
2. Thyroid function tests
3. Stool studies if malabsorption suspected
4. Chest X-ray if respiratory symptoms present
5. Referral for specialized tests as indicated

Differential Diagnosis

1. Inadequate caloric intake (neglect, feeding difficulties)
2. Malabsorption syndromes (celiac disease, cystic fibrosis)
3. Chronic infections (TB, HIV)
4. Congenital heart disease
5. Metabolic or endocrine disorders

Management in the Rural Setting

1. Provide nutritional counseling and education to caregivers
2. Treat underlying diseases and infections
3. Coordinate with social services and community resources
4. Monitor growth parameters regularly
5. Refer to pediatric specialists for complex cases

Disposition and Transfer Criteria

1. Transfer if severe malnutrition with complications
2. Transfer if underlying serious medical condition identified
3. Admit locally if stable and plan for outpatient follow-up
4. Urgent referral if developmental delay or failure to respond to initial management

Parental Communication & Reassurance

1. Educate on importance of nutrition and feeding practices
2. Provide support and resources for families
3. Explain the evaluation process and need for follow-up
4. Encourage positive caregiver-child interaction

Documentation Essentials

1. Growth measurements and trends
2. Feeding history and dietary intake
3. Physical exam findings
4. Investigations and results
5. Communication and referral notes

Practical Pearls for Rural Docs

1. Growth charts are essential tools for early detection
2. Consider social determinants of health in assessment
3. Early intervention can prevent long-term consequences
4. Collaborate with multidisciplinary teams for best outcomes

CHAPTER 16:
Febrile Seizures

Overview

Febrile seizures are the most common type of seizure in children aged 6 months to 5 years. They occur in the setting of fever without evidence of CNS infection or other underlying neurologic disorder. They are categorized as simple (generalized, <15 minutes, single episode in 24h) or complex (focal, prolonged, or recurrent).

Red Flags – "Don't Miss" Features

1. Seizure >15 minutes or multiple seizures within 24 hours
2. Focal seizure features (e.g., one-sided twitching)
3. Signs of meningitis: neck stiffness, photophobia, bulging fontanelle
4. Persistent altered consciousness post-seizure
5. Age <6 months or >5 years

Initial Assessment in the Rural ER

1. ABCs: ensure airway, breathing, and circulation are stable
2. Check blood glucose immediately
3. Obtain a thorough history: fever onset, duration, seizure characteristics, past history
4. Assess for signs of CNS infection or trauma

Stabilization Protocol

1. Ensure airway is patent; suction and oxygen if needed
2. Administer antipyretics (acetaminophen 15 mg/kg PO/PR or ibuprofen 10 mg/kg PO)
3. If seizure ongoing >5 minutes, treat as status epilepticus (e.g., lorazepam 0.1 mg/kg IV)

4. Monitor vital signs and neurological status

Investigations

1. **Simple febrile seizure**: No labs or imaging typically required
2. **Complex or atypical features**:
3. CBC, electrolytes, glucose
4. Blood culture if ill-appearing
5. Consider LP if <12 months and not immunized or showing meningeal signs
6. CT head if focal features or signs of increased ICP

Differential Diagnosis

1. Meningitis / Encephalitis
2. Epilepsy
3. Metabolic abnormalities (e.g., hyponatremia, hypoglycemia)
4. Febrile seizure (simple vs complex)
5. Trauma / non-accidental injury

Management in the Rural Setting

1. Reassure parents if seizure is simple and resolved
2. Treat fever and provide hydration
3. Educate about recurrence risk (25–30%) and good prognosis
4. Observe in ER for several hours if first episode or complex features

Disposition and Transfer Criteria

1. **Safe for discharge** if simple febrile seizure, child is well-appearing, and no red flags

Transfer if:

1. Complex febrile seizure
2. Prolonged postictal phase or focal deficits
3. Suspicion of CNS infection or trauma
4. Infant <6 months or ill-appearing child

Parental Communication & Reassurance

1. Explain that febrile seizures are common and generally benign
2. Provide fever management plan
3. Discuss recurrence risk and when to return to ER
4. Advise against home use of antiepileptics unless prescribed by pediatric neurologist

Documentation Essentials

1. Description of seizure: duration, focality, number
2. Vital signs and fever documentation
3. Neurological exam post-event
4. Parental discussion and discharge/transfer plans

Practical Pearls for Rural Docs

1. Febrile seizures rarely cause long-term harm
2. Avoid unnecessary investigations in classic simple febrile seizures
3. Always rule out CNS infection in complex or atypical cases
4. Use age-appropriate fever thresholds and dosing

CHAPTER 17:
Fluid Resuscitation in Children

Overview

Fluid resuscitation in children is a critical intervention for shock, dehydration, and volume depletion. Pediatric patients have unique physiological considerations requiring careful assessment and weight-based fluid administration to restore perfusion and prevent complications.

Red Flags – "Don't Miss" Features

1. Signs of shock: tachycardia, delayed capillary refill, hypotension (late sign)
2. Altered mental status or lethargy
3. Poor urine output or anuria
4. Signs of dehydration (dry mucous membranes, sunken eyes)
5. Cool extremities and weak pulses

Initial Assessment in the Rural ER

1. Assess airway, breathing, and circulation
2. Measure vital signs including heart rate, blood pressure, respiratory rate
3. Evaluate hydration status and level of consciousness
4. Determine weight for fluid calculations
5. Obtain history of fluid losses and illness duration

Stabilization Protocol

1. Establish vascular access (IV or IO)
2. Administer isotonic crystalloid boluses (20 mL/kg over 10–20 minutes)
3. Repeat boluses as needed, up to 60 mL/kg initially

4. Monitor response: heart rate, perfusion, mental status, urine output
5. Avoid fluid overload, especially in cardiac or renal disease

Investigations

1. Blood glucose to rule out hypoglycemia
2. Electrolytes, BUN, creatinine
3. Blood gas analysis if acid-base disturbances suspected
4. CBC and lactate in sepsis or shock

Differential Diagnosis

1. Hypovolemic shock due to dehydration or hemorrhage
2. Septic shock
3. Cardiogenic shock
4. Distributive shock (anaphylaxis, neurogenic)

Management in the Rural Setting

1. Rapid recognition and treatment of shock
2. Use weight-based dosing for fluid administration
3. Monitor closely for signs of fluid overload or pulmonary edema
4. Provide supportive care including oxygen and temperature control
5. Prepare for urgent transfer if unstable or requiring advanced care

Disposition and Transfer Criteria

1. Transfer if persistent shock despite fluid resuscitation
2. Transfer for respiratory distress or multi-organ failure
3. Admit locally if stable with ongoing monitoring
4. Communicate fluid management details during transfer

Parental Communication & Reassurance

1. Explain importance of fluids and monitoring
2. Reassure on treatment goals and expected improvement
3. Provide guidance on warning signs and when to seek help

Documentation Essentials

1. Fluid volumes and timing
2. Patient response and vital signs
3. Vascular access sites and complications
4. Communication with family and receiving team

Practical Pearls for Rural Docs

1. Start fluid resuscitation promptly in shock states
2. Use isotonic fluids, avoid hypotonic solutions
3. Monitor for signs of overload, especially in infants and cardiac patients
4. Adjust fluid rates based on ongoing assessment

CHAPTER 18:
Foreign Body Aspiration

Overview

Foreign body aspiration (FBA) is a potentially life-threatening emergency in children, especially those aged 6 months to 4 years. It typically involves sudden onset coughing, choking, or wheezing after eating or playing. Organic materials (nuts, seeds) are most common. Diagnosis may be missed if the event is unwitnessed. Early recognition and airway management are critical.

Red Flags – "Don't Miss" Features

1. Sudden onset of cough, gagging, or choking during eating or play
2. Unilateral wheezing or decreased breath sounds
3. Persistent cough not responding to bronchodilators
4. Cyanosis, respiratory distress, or stridor
5. History suggestive of aspiration without resolution

Initial Assessment in the Rural ER

1. ABCs and vital signs (look for signs of hypoxia or distress)
2. History from caregiver: what was the child doing, eating, or playing with?
3. Assess airway patency, work of breathing, oxygen saturation
4. Auscultation: localized wheezing, decreased air entry, or asymmetry
5. Look for signs of upper vs lower airway obstruction

Stabilization Protocol

If complete obstruction (unable to cough or speak):

1. Infants <1 year: 5 back blows + 5 chest thrusts
2. Children >1 year: Heimlich maneuver (abdominal thrusts)
3. Call for help immediately if no response

If partial obstruction (coughing, breathing):

1. Keep child calm and in position of comfort
2. Administer oxygen and monitor closely
3. Avoid blind finger sweeps or attempts to remove object without visualization
4. Prepare for deterioration and potential need for intubation

Investigations

1. Chest and neck X-rays (inspiratory and expiratory views if possible)
2. Look for air trapping, atelectasis, or radiopaque object
3. Normal imaging does not rule out FBA
4. Rigid bronchoscopy is gold standard for diagnosis and removal

Differential Diagnosis

1. Foreign body aspiration (upper or lower airway)
2. Asthma or bronchiolitis
3. Croup or epiglottitis
4. Anaphylaxis or airway edema
5. Pneumonia or atelectasis

Management in the Rural Setting

1. Stabilize airway and breathing
2. Administer supplemental oxygen
3. Avoid unnecessary sedation or interventions unless airway is threatened
4. If object is visible and easily accessible in oropharynx, remove gently
5. Consult pediatric ENT or anesthesia if advanced airway needed
6. Do not delay transfer for bronchoscopy if FBA suspected

Disposition and Transfer Criteria

Transfer urgently if:

1. Any signs of persistent obstruction or distress
2. Suspected lower airway foreign body even if stable
3. Need for bronchoscopy (diagnostic and therapeutic)
4. Unwitnessed episode with persistent respiratory findings
5. **Discharge** only if: well-appearing, normal auscultation, clear history, and normal imaging (if obtained)

Parental Communication & Reassurance

1. Explain the seriousness and risk of recurrence
2. Recommend food safety for young children (avoid nuts, hard candy)
3. Provide return precautions (wheezing, cough, fever, difficulty breathing)
4. Reinforce importance of supervision during meals and play

Documentation Essentials

1. Time and nature of choking episode
2. Airway status on arrival and during stay
3. Interventions performed (e.g., back blows, Heimlich)

4. Imaging results, consultations, and disposition plan

Practical Pearls for Rural Docs

1. Always suspect FBA in a previously well child with sudden respiratory symptoms
2. Normal chest X-ray does not exclude foreign body—history is key
3. Unilateral wheeze or air trapping = high suspicion for FBA
4. Don't delay transfer for bronchoscopy if high-risk features present

CHAPTER 19:
Fractures in Children (Supracondylar, Greenstick)

Overview

Fractures in children are common injuries, with supracondylar humerus fractures and greenstick fractures being among the most frequent. These fractures have unique pediatric considerations, including growth plate involvement, and require careful assessment to prevent complications like neurovascular injury or malunion.

Red Flags – "Don't Miss" Features

1. Swelling, deformity, and tenderness at fracture site
2. Neurovascular compromise (absent pulses, pallor, paresthesia)
3. Open fractures or skin breach
4. Severe pain unrelieved by analgesia
5. Compartment syndrome signs (pain out of proportion, paralysis)
6. Limited range of motion or severe angulation

Initial Assessment in the Rural ER

1. Assess ABCs and stabilize patient if polytrauma
2. Inspect limb for deformity, swelling, wounds
3. Check distal pulses and capillary refill
4. Assess motor and sensory function distal to injury
5. Obtain history of mechanism and timing of injury

Stabilization Protocol

1. Immobilize limb with appropriate splint or sling
2. Elevate injured limb and apply ice packs to reduce swelling

3. Administer analgesics as needed (weight-based dosing)
4. Monitor neurovascular status frequently
5. Prepare for timely transfer if unstable or complicated fracture

Investigations

1. Obtain X-rays of the affected limb in two planes
2. Assess for involvement of growth plate (Salter-Harris classification)
3. Imaging of adjacent joints if indicated
4. Ultrasound or Doppler if vascular injury suspected

Differential Diagnosis

1. Fracture (supracondylar, greenstick, buckle)
2. Sprain or ligamentous injury
3. Contusion or soft tissue injury
4. Infection (osteomyelitis)
5. Non-accidental trauma in suspicious cases

Management in the Rural Setting

1. Provide pain control and immobilize promptly
2. Reduce displaced supracondylar fractures only if trained and stable
3. Urgent transfer if neurovascular compromise or open fracture
4. Educate caregivers about splint care and follow-up
5. Arrange orthopedic consultation for definitive management

Disposition and Transfer Criteria

Transfer urgently if:

1. Open fractures
2. Neurovascular compromise
3. Significant displacement requiring reduction

4. Signs of compartment syndrome
5. Discharge if minor buckle fractures and stable with splint and analgesia

Parental Communication & Reassurance

1. Explain nature of fracture and need for immobilization
2. Discuss expected healing and follow-up plans
3. Educate on signs of worsening neurovascular status or pain
4. Provide instructions for splint care and activity restrictions

Documentation Essentials

1. Detailed neurovascular exam findings
2. Description of deformity and swelling
3. Analgesia given and response
4. Imaging reports and plans for referral or transfer

Practical Pearls for Rural Docs

1. Supracondylar fractures are associated with risk of Volkmann's ischemic contracture—monitor pulses closely
2. Greenstick fractures may be stable but require orthopedic follow-up
3. Always check neurovascular status before and after any manipulation
4. Immobilize in position of comfort and avoid unnecessary movement

CHAPTER 20:
Head Trauma – Concussion, Skull Fracture, Intracranial Bleeds

Overview

Head trauma is a common pediatric presentation in rural ERs, ranging from mild concussions to life-threatening skull fractures and intracranial bleeds. Children are particularly vulnerable due to anatomical differences (larger head-to-body ratio, thinner skull). Early recognition of red flags and appropriate imaging/transfer decisions are key.

Red Flags – "Don't Miss" Features

1. GCS <15 or any decline in mental status
2. Vomiting ≥2 times post-head injury
3. Seizure or post-traumatic amnesia
4. Focal neurologic deficits
5. Signs of skull fracture (raccoon eyes, Battle sign, CSF leak from nose/ear)
6. Bulging fontanelle (infants)
7. Irritability or altered behaviour not improving
8. Mechanism: fall >1 meter (infants), >1.5 meters (older kids), MVA, or abuse

Initial Assessment in the Rural ER

1. ABCs: secure airway if GCS <8, assess oxygenation and perfusion
2. Full GCS scoring, pupil reaction, vital signs
3. History: LOC, seizure, vomiting, amnesia, mechanism
4. Physical exam: scalp lacerations, hematoma, signs of basilar skull fracture

5. Consider cervical spine precautions if high-impact mechanism

Stabilization Protocol

1. Maintain airway and oxygenation; intubate if GCS ≤8
2. Immobilize cervical spine if indicated
3. Control bleeding with pressure or dressing
4. IV access, isotonic fluids if hypotensive
5. Treat seizures with lorazepam 0.1 mg/kg IV
6. Avoid hypotension and hypoxia – both worsen outcomes in TBI

Investigations

1. Glucose, CBC, electrolytes
2. CT head (non-contrast) is the gold standard if red flags present
3. Avoid routine CT in low-risk kids (use PECARN decision rule)
4. C-spine x-ray if neck pain or mechanism warrants
5. Monitor vital signs and neurologic status over time

Differential Diagnosis

1. Concussion (mild TBI)
2. Epidural hematoma (lucid interval, rapid deterioration)
3. Subdural hematoma (gradual LOC decline, shaken baby syndrome)
4. Skull fracture (depressed or basilar)
5. Scalp hematoma (cephalohematoma, subgaleal bleed)
6. Non-accidental injury (consider in infants or unusual presentation)

Management in the Rural Setting

1. **Concussion**: Rest, hydration, avoid screens, no return to sport/school until full recovery; educate parents
2. **Skull fracture or bleed**: Stabilize and transfer urgently

3. Administer analgesia carefully (avoid oversedation)
4. Monitor GCS hourly if staying in rural facility temporarily

Disposition and Transfer Criteria

1. **Discharge if**: isolated concussion, normal neuro exam, no red flags, reliable parents

Transfer if:

1. GCS <15 or decline during observation
2. Seizure, persistent vomiting, focal deficits
3. CT shows fracture or bleed
4. Suspected abusive head trauma
5. Call receiving pediatric trauma/neurosurgery team early

Parental Communication & Reassurance

1. Clearly explain red flags to monitor at home (vomiting, drowsiness, confusion)
2. Emphasize no sports or strenuous activity until cleared
3. Give written head injury advice sheet if discharging
4. Discuss need for follow-up if symptoms persist >1 week

Documentation Essentials

1. Mechanism of injury and history from caregivers
2. Neurological exam and GCS at each reassessment
3. CT findings or reason for not imaging (PECARN rule)
4. Parental discussion and discharge/transfer details

Practical Pearls for Rural Docs

1. Use PECARN rule to minimize unnecessary CT scans
2. Vomiting alone is not always an indication for CT but needs context

3. Always consider non-accidental injury in infants or unwitnessed trauma
4. Don't miss lucid interval in epidural hematoma – deterioration can be rapid

CHAPTER 21:
Headache – Emergency vs Benign

Overview

Headache is a common pediatric complaint and often benign, but in emergency settings, it is crucial to rule out life-threatening causes such as meningitis, intracranial hemorrhage, or mass effect. A focused history and neurologic exam can help distinguish primary from secondary headaches, guiding safe rural management or urgent transfer.

Red Flags – "Don't Miss" Features

1. Sudden onset "thunderclap" headache
2. Severe headache with altered mental status or seizure
3. Fever, neck stiffness, photophobia (meningitis concern)
4. Focal neurologic deficits (e.g., diplopia, weakness, ataxia)
5. Papilledema or signs of increased intracranial pressure
6. Worsening headache over days, especially with vomiting
7. Headache waking child from sleep or worse in morning
8. Recent head trauma or anticoagulant use

Initial Assessment in the Rural ER

1. Assess ABCs and vital signs
2. Detailed history: onset, duration, severity, pattern, triggers
3. Inquire about recent infections, trauma, visual changes, or school stress
4. Perform full neurologic exam including fundoscopic exam (if possible)
5. Check hydration status and signs of systemic illness

Stabilization Protocol

1. Ensure patient comfort and dark/quiet environment
2. Treat nausea and pain with age-appropriate medications (e.g., acetaminophen, ibuprofen, ondansetron)
3. Administer IV fluids if dehydrated or vomiting
4. Prepare for imaging or transfer if red flags present
5. Avoid narcotics for primary headache

Investigations

1. None required for typical, recurrent benign headache
2. CT head if red flags (e.g., focal signs, altered LOC, papilledema)
3. LP if meningitis or idiopathic intracranial hypertension suspected (after CT if needed)
4. CBC and CRP if infection suspected
5. Urine tox screen in adolescent with atypical presentation

Differential Diagnosis

1. Primary headaches: migraine, tension-type, cluster (rare in children)
2. Post-viral headache
3. Meningitis or encephalitis
4. Intracranial mass or hydrocephalus
5. Idiopathic intracranial hypertension (especially in obese adolescents)
6. Trauma-related (e.g., subdural hematoma)
7. Sinusitis-related headache

Management in the Rural Setting

1. Manage pain with acetaminophen or ibuprofen
2. Consider oral triptans in adolescents with known migraines
3. Use antiemetics (e.g., ondansetron) for migraine-associated nausea

4. Rehydrate if dehydrated or vomiting
5. Reassure if no red flags and consistent with primary headache
6. Plan for outpatient neurology follow-up if recurrent or impairing function

Disposition and Transfer Criteria

1. Urgent transfer if red flags: altered mental status, focal signs, signs of raised ICP
2. Transfer if CT or LP not available and serious pathology suspected
3. Discharge with follow-up if stable, well-appearing, and consistent with primary headache

Parental Communication & Reassurance

1. Explain the difference between primary and concerning headaches
2. Provide guidance on hydration, regular meals, and sleep hygiene
3. Reinforce red flags that warrant return to hospital (vomiting, confusion, persistent pain)
4. Discuss need for follow-up if recurrent or school-limiting

Documentation Essentials

1. Detailed history of headache characteristics and associated symptoms
2. Neurologic and general physical exam findings
3. Any imaging or labs ordered
4. Response to analgesia and hydration
5. Disposition plan and parental instructions

Practical Pearls for Rural Docs

1. Thunderclap headache, focal signs, or papilledema always warrant imaging
2. Recurrent headaches with normal exam are usually benign
3. Sinus headaches are often overdiagnosed – rule out other causes
4. In infants, consider bulging fontanelle or irritability as clues to ICP

Avoid overuse of imaging in children with typical migraine patterns

CHAPTER 22:
IV Access – IO Access in Emergencies

Overview

Establishing vascular access in pediatric emergencies is critical for fluid resuscitation, medication administration, and blood sampling. Intraosseous (IO) access provides a rapid alternative when intravenous (IV) access is difficult or delayed, especially in critically ill children.

Red Flags – "Don't Miss" Features

1. Difficulty or delay in obtaining peripheral IV access
2. Need for rapid fluid or medication administration
3. Signs of shock or poor perfusion
4. Cardiac arrest or respiratory failure requiring immediate access
5. Severe dehydration or collapsed veins

Initial Assessment in the Rural ER

1. Assess the child's condition and urgency of access
2. Attempt peripheral IV access in appropriate sites
3. Consider central access if skilled and time permits
4. Prepare equipment for IO access if IV unsuccessful or time-critical

Stabilization Protocol

1. Use topical anesthetic or sedation if possible for IV attempts
2. Follow aseptic technique for insertion
3. For IO access, select appropriate site (proximal tibia, distal femur, humerus)
4. Secure IO needle properly to prevent dislodgement
5. Monitor insertion site for complications

Investigations

1. Not applicable for access itself, but verify placement by:
2. Aspiration of marrow or blood
3. Ability to flush without resistance
4. Response to fluid bolus or medications

Differential Diagnosis

1. Peripheral IV access feasible
2. Central venous access indicated
3. IO access for emergency situations

Management in the Rural Setting

1. Train staff in IO insertion techniques
2. Have IO kits readily available in emergency settings
3. Prioritize IO access if IV attempts fail after 1–2 tries or 90 seconds
4. Use IO for fluid resuscitation, drug delivery, and blood sampling
5. Remove IO access within 24 hours and replace with IV when stable

Disposition and Transfer Criteria

1. Transfer if patient remains unstable or requires advanced care
2. Ensure vascular access is maintained during transfer
3. Communicate access details to receiving team

Parental Communication & Reassurance

1. Explain the need for rapid access and methods used
2. Reassure about safety and temporary nature of IO access
3. Address pain or discomfort and provide support

Documentation Essentials

1. Time, site, and method of vascular access
2. Number of attempts and success/failure
3. Medications and fluids administered via access
4. Complications or difficulties encountered

Practical Pearls for Rural Docs

1. IO access is a lifesaving alternative when IV access fails
2. Familiarize with anatomical landmarks and devices
3. Practice aseptic technique to minimize infection risk
4. Monitor for extravasation or compartment syndrome

CHAPTER 23:
Incarcerated Hernia

Overview

Incarcerated hernia is a surgical emergency where herniated bowel or tissue becomes trapped and cannot be reduced, risking ischemia and strangulation. Early recognition and prompt surgical referral are critical in pediatric patients.

Red Flags – "Don't Miss" Features

1. Irreducible, tender groin or scrotal swelling
2. Abdominal distension or vomiting
3. Signs of bowel obstruction or ischemia
4. Fever or systemic toxicity
5. Skin changes over hernia site (erythema, discoloration)

Initial Assessment in the Rural ER

1. Assess ABCs and vital signs
2. Examine groin and scrotum for swelling, tenderness, and color changes
3. Assess for signs of bowel obstruction
4. Obtain history of onset, duration, and reducibility
5. Monitor hydration and pain level

Stabilization Protocol

1. Provide analgesia and antiemetics as needed
2. Attempt gentle manual reduction only if no signs of strangulation and trained to do so
3. Establish IV access and start fluids if vomiting or dehydrated
4. Prepare for urgent surgical transfer if reduction unsuccessful or signs of ischemia present

Investigations

1. Abdominal x-ray if bowel obstruction suspected
2. Ultrasound to assess bowel viability if available
3. Laboratory tests if systemic illness present

Differential Diagnosis

1. Inguinal hernia (reducible)
2. Hydrocele
3. Testicular torsion
4. Lymphadenopathy
5. Abscess

Management in the Rural Setting

1. Stabilize patient and assess need for manual reduction
2. Do not delay transfer if strangulation suspected
3. Provide supportive care and analgesia
4. Communicate with surgical team early for transfer planning

Disposition and Transfer Criteria

1. Urgent transfer for suspected strangulated hernia
2. Admit locally if successful reduction and stable
3. Monitor for signs of recurrence or complications

Parental Communication & Reassurance

1. Explain urgency of condition and treatment plan
2. Educate about signs of complications and recurrence
3. Reassure regarding surgical treatment outcomes

Documentation Essentials

1. Hernia characteristics and reduction attempts
2. Vital signs and hydration status
3. Imaging and lab results
4. Transfer communication and plans

Practical Pearls for Rural Docs

1. Avoid forceful reduction attempts to prevent injury
2. Manual reduction can be successful if done early and gently
3. Early surgical consultation improves outcomes
4. Monitor closely for signs of bowel ischemia

CHAPTER 24:
Insect Bites

Overview

Insect bites are common in children and can cause localized reactions, allergic responses, or rarely systemic illness. Rural providers should recognize signs of severe allergic reactions, secondary infections, and appropriate treatment strategies.

Red Flags – "Don't Miss" Features

1. Severe allergic reaction or anaphylaxis
2. Extensive swelling, erythema, or cellulitis
3. Signs of systemic infection: fever, malaise
4. Bite in sensitive areas (face, eyes, genitals)
5. Suspected venomous bites or stings

Initial Assessment in the Rural ER

1. Assess airway, breathing, circulation
2. Obtain history of bite/sting, timing, and insect type if known
3. Examine bite site for swelling, redness, necrosis, or signs of infection
4. Monitor vital signs and allergic symptoms
5. Assess for pain and functional impairment

Stabilization Protocol

1. Manage anaphylaxis with IM epinephrine immediately if present
2. Provide analgesia and antihistamines for mild reactions
3. Clean wound and apply cold compresses
4. Initiate antibiotics if secondary infection suspected
5. Observe for progression of swelling or systemic symptoms

Investigations

1. Clinical diagnosis in most cases
2. Wound cultures if infection suspected
3. Blood tests if systemic symptoms present
4. Imaging if deep tissue involvement or retained foreign body

Differential Diagnosis

1. Allergic reaction to insect bite or sting
2. Cellulitis or abscess
3. Other dermatologic conditions (eczema, contact dermatitis)
4. Tick-borne illnesses (Lyme disease, Rocky Mountain spotted fever)
5. Spider bites or venomous arthropod envenomation

Management in the Rural Setting

1. Provide symptomatic treatment and wound care
2. Educate caregivers on bite prevention and signs of complications
3. Initiate prompt treatment for allergic reactions or infections
4. Arrange transfer if severe systemic involvement or envenomation suspected

Disposition and Transfer Criteria

1. Transfer if anaphylaxis or severe systemic reaction
2. Transfer if spreading cellulitis or deep tissue infection
3. Discharge with follow-up for mild localized reactions

Parental Communication & Reassurance

1. Reassure about common mild reactions and self-limited course
2. Educate on when to seek urgent care (breathing difficulty, swelling)

3. Provide instructions on wound care and symptom monitoring
4. Discuss preventive measures like insect repellents and protective clothing

Documentation Essentials

1. Description of bite/sting site and symptoms
2. Treatments given and patient response
3. Allergic reactions and interventions
4. Communication with family and follow-up plan

Practical Pearls for Rural Docs

1. Early recognition of anaphylaxis saves lives
2. Secondary infections are common; treat promptly
3. Venomous bites require specialist consultation
4. Always provide thorough education and follow-up instructions

CHAPTER 25:
Intussusception

Overview

Intussusception is the telescoping of one segment of bowel into another, leading to obstruction and ischemia. It commonly affects infants 6 months to 2 years old and presents with episodic abdominal pain, vomiting, and bloody stools. Timely diagnosis and treatment prevent complications.

Red Flags – "Don't Miss" Features

1. Sudden, severe intermittent abdominal pain
2. Vomiting, sometimes bilious
3. "Currant jelly" stools (blood and mucus)
4. Abdominal distension or palpable sausage-shaped mass
5. Lethargy or signs of shock

Initial Assessment in the Rural ER

1. Assess ABCs and hydration status
2. Obtain detailed history of pain episodes and stool characteristics
3. Examine abdomen for distension, tenderness, and mass
4. Monitor vital signs and neurological status

Stabilization Protocol

1. Initiate IV fluids for dehydration
2. Provide analgesia judiciously
3. Prepare for possible nasogastric decompression
4. Arrange urgent transfer for diagnostic imaging and reduction

Investigations

1. Abdominal ultrasound is diagnostic (target or doughnut sign)
2. Abdominal x-ray may show obstruction or soft tissue mass
3. CBC and electrolytes to assess hydration and infection

Differential Diagnosis

1. Gastroenteritis
2. Appendicitis
3. Intestinal obstruction from other causes
4. Hirschsprung disease
5. Meckel diverticulum

Management in the Rural Setting

1. Supportive care with fluids and pain control
2. Do not attempt reduction unless skilled and equipped
3. Arrange urgent transfer to tertiary center for imaging and enema reduction
4. Monitor for signs of bowel perforation or peritonitis

Disposition and Transfer Criteria

1. Urgent transfer for all suspected cases
2. Stabilize and prepare for transport
3. Notify receiving center of clinical status and interventions

Parental Communication & Reassurance

1. Explain the nature and urgency of the condition
2. Discuss signs to monitor and need for hospital care
3. Reassure about generally good outcomes with prompt treatment

Documentation Essentials

1. Description of pain episodes and stool findings
2. Physical exam and vital signs
3. Fluids administered and response
4. Communication and transfer details

Practical Pearls for Rural Docs

1. Intussusception is the most common cause of bowel obstruction in infants
2. Ultrasound is highly sensitive and specific for diagnosis
3. Early transfer reduces risk of bowel necrosis and surgery
4. Be alert for intermittent symptoms and "normal" exams between episodes

CHAPTER 26:
Meningitis & Encephalitis

Overview

Meningitis is inflammation of the meninges, while encephalitis involves inflammation of the brain parenchyma. Both conditions are medical emergencies, particularly in children. Bacterial meningitis can progress rapidly and is associated with high morbidity and mortality if untreated. Viral causes (e.g., HSV, enteroviruses) are more common in encephalitis.

Red Flags – "Don't Miss" Features

1. Fever with altered mental status
2. Bulging fontanelle (infants), neck stiffness (older children)
3. Seizures (especially new onset or focal)
4. Petechial or purpuric rash (meningococcemia)
5. Vomiting, photophobia, severe headache
6. Hypotension, poor perfusion, lethargy

Initial Assessment in the Rural ER

1. ABCs: airway protection if altered LOC or seizures
2. Full vital signs and blood glucose
3. Assess mental status: irritability, lethargy, confusion
4. Fontanelle exam in infants; Kernig and Brudzinski signs in older children
5. Identify signs of increased ICP or sepsis

Stabilization Protocol

1. Secure airway if GCS ≤8 or evidence of poor respiratory effort
2. Administer oxygen and IV fluids (isotonic bolus 20 mL/kg if hypotensive)

3. Begin empiric IV antibiotics ASAP after cultures:
4. <1 month: Ampicillin + Cefotaxime ± Acyclovir
5. ≥1 month: Ceftriaxone 100 mg/kg/day + Vancomycin 60 mg/kg/day divided q6h ± Acyclovir 20 mg/kg IV q8h
6. Manage seizures if present (e.g., lorazepam, fosphenytoin)
7. Elevate head of bed, avoid fluid overload if ↑ICP suspected

Investigations

1. CBC, electrolytes, glucose, CRP
2. Blood cultures x2
3. LP (after CT if indicated): opening pressure, cell count, glucose, protein, Gram stain, culture, PCR
4. CT head before LP if: focal deficits, papilledema, severe altered LOC
5. HSV PCR from CSF if encephalitis suspected

Differential Diagnosis

1. Bacterial meningitis (Neisseria, Strep pneumo, GBS)
2. Viral encephalitis (HSV, enterovirus, arboviruses)
3. Sepsis with altered mental status
4. Brain abscess or tumor
5. Non-infectious causes: ADEM, autoimmune encephalitis, toxins

Management in the Rural Setting

1. Early recognition and empiric treatment are critical
2. Give antibiotics before LP if delay or instability
3. Acyclovir if any suspicion of HSV (encephalitis, temporal lobe signs, seizures)
4. Isolate until meningitis type confirmed (droplet precautions)
5. Consult pediatric infectious diseases or tertiary center early

Disposition and Transfer Criteria

1. **Urgent transfer** required in nearly all cases
2. Stabilize airway and hemodynamics before transfer
3. Continuous monitoring during transport
4. Discuss with pediatric ICU or tertiary infectious disease service prior to departure

Parental Communication & Reassurance

1. Explain seriousness and need for urgent treatment and transfer
2. Reassure that early treatment can be lifesaving
3. Provide infection control information (e.g., prophylaxis for contacts in meningococcal disease)
4. Discuss expected investigations and hospitalization

Documentation Essentials

1. Onset and description of symptoms (fever, seizures, LOC)
2. Vital signs and physical exam findings (fontanelle, neck stiffness)
3. Medications and doses given (antibiotics, antivirals, antiepileptics)
4. Parental discussions and consent for transfer

Practical Pearls for Rural Docs

1. Never delay antibiotics for imaging or LP in unstable patients
2. Consider HSV in neonates, altered LOC, focal seizures
3. Always dose antibiotics and antivirals based on weight
4. Don't forget glucose before LP—hypoglycemia can mimic meningitis

CHAPTER 27:
Neck Injuries – C-spine Clearance in Children

Overview

Cervical spine injuries in children require careful assessment due to anatomical and developmental differences compared to adults. Proper clearance of the C-spine is crucial to avoid missing unstable injuries. Rural providers should follow pediatric-specific criteria to decide when imaging or immobilization is needed.

Red Flags – "Don't Miss" Features

1. Neck pain or tenderness after trauma
2. Neurological deficits: weakness, numbness, paralysis
3. Altered level of consciousness
4. Significant mechanism of injury (high-speed MVC, fall from height)
5. Presence of distracting injuries
6. Signs of spinal cord injury: hypotonia, areflexia, loss of bladder/bowel control

Initial Assessment in the Rural ER

1. Conduct ABCs and stabilize patient
2. Assess airway while maintaining cervical spine precautions
3. Detailed neurological examination focusing on motor and sensory function
4. Evaluate neck range of motion cautiously
5. Obtain history regarding mechanism and symptoms

Stabilization Protocol

1. Maintain in-line cervical spine immobilization with collar or manual stabilization
2. Provide oxygen and support breathing as needed
3. Establish IV access for fluids and medications
4. Monitor vital signs and neurological status frequently
5. Avoid unnecessary movement or manipulation of neck

Investigations

1. Use pediatric-specific clinical decision rules (e.g., NEXUS, PECARN) for imaging
2. Lateral cervical spine X-ray in 3 views (AP, lateral, odontoid) if indicated
3. CT cervical spine if X-rays inconclusive and suspicion remains high
4. MRI if neurological deficits or cord injury suspected

Differential Diagnosis

1. Cervical spine fracture or dislocation
2. Ligamentous injury or sprain
3. Spinal cord injury without radiographic abnormality (SCIWORA)
4. Muscle strain or soft tissue injury
5. Congenital cervical anomalies

Management in the Rural Setting

1. Immobilize cervical spine if injury suspected or unclear
2. Use appropriate-sized cervical collars for children
3. Initiate prompt transfer to trauma or neurosurgical center if unstable or neurological deficit present
4. Provide analgesia and monitor for deterioration
5. Avoid premature collar removal before clearance

Disposition and Transfer Criteria

Transfer urgently if:

1. Unstable cervical spine injury or fracture
2. Neurological deficits
3. High-risk mechanism with uncertain imaging
4. Local observation only if low-risk and fully cleared clinically and radiographically

Parental Communication & Reassurance

1. Explain need for neck immobilization and possible imaging
2. Reassure that careful assessment minimizes risk of missed injury
3. Discuss transfer reasons if needed and expected course
4. Provide instructions on immobilization and activity restrictions

Documentation Essentials

1. Neurological exam findings
2. Details of mechanism of injury
3. Imaging performed and results
4. Neck immobilization method and duration
5. Communication with family and transfer plans

Practical Pearls for Rural Docs

1. Pediatric neck anatomy differs: increased ligamentous laxity and larger head size increase risk
2. SCIWORA can occur despite normal X-rays; consider MRI if neurological signs present
3. Use PECARN or NEXUS rules tailored for children to avoid unnecessary imaging
4. Always maintain immobilization until definitive clearance

CHAPTER 28:
Neonatal Jaundice – Severe Hyperbilirubinemia

Overview

Neonatal jaundice is common, but severe hyperbilirubinemia can cause kernicterus and irreversible neurological damage. Early recognition, risk stratification, and timely treatment such as phototherapy or exchange transfusion are essential in rural settings.

Red Flags – "Don't Miss" Features

1. Jaundice appearing within 24 hours of life
2. Rapidly rising bilirubin levels
3. Poor feeding or lethargy
4. High-pitched crying or irritability
5. Arching of the neck and body (opisthotonos)
6. Hypotonia or seizures
7. Dark urine and pale stools

Initial Assessment in the Rural ER

1. Assess general appearance and hydration status
2. Measure vital signs
3. Perform a careful physical exam to confirm jaundice and neurological signs
4. Obtain history of birth, feeding, family history of hemolysis or jaundice
5. Evaluate risk factors such as prematurity or blood group incompatibility

Stabilization Protocol

1. Ensure adequate hydration and feeding support
2. Initiate phototherapy if bilirubin above treatment thresholds
3. Prepare for exchange transfusion in severe or rapidly rising cases
4. Monitor vital signs and neurological status closely
5. Consult pediatric specialists early for management guidance

Investigations

1. Total and direct serum bilirubin levels
2. Blood group and Coombs test (direct antiglobulin test)
3. CBC and reticulocyte count
4. Liver function tests
5. Blood smear if hemolysis suspected

Differential Diagnosis

1. Physiologic jaundice of the newborn
2. Hemolytic disease of the newborn (ABO or Rh incompatibility)
3. Infection (sepsis)
4. Metabolic disorders (e.g., G6PD deficiency)
5. Biliary atresia or liver disease

Management in the Rural Setting

1. Start phototherapy promptly based on bilirubin levels and age in hours
2. Maintain feeding and hydration
3. Monitor bilirubin trends and clinical status
4. Arrange urgent transfer for exchange transfusion if indicated
5. Educate parents about signs of worsening jaundice

Disposition and Transfer Criteria

Transfer if:

1. Bilirubin exceeds exchange transfusion threshold
2. Signs of acute bilirubin encephalopathy
3. Poor feeding, lethargy, or seizures present
4. Unable to provide intensive phototherapy locally

Parental Communication & Reassurance

1. Explain cause of jaundice and treatment options
2. Reassure about prognosis with timely treatment
3. Instruct on feeding, hydration, and recognizing worsening signs
4. Provide clear follow-up instructions

Documentation Essentials

1. Bilirubin levels and trend
2. Physical exam findings, including neurological status
3. Treatments given (phototherapy, transfusion)
4. Parental discussions and transfer plan

Practical Pearls for Rural Docs

1. Early jaundice (within 24h) is always concerning
2. Use age-specific bilirubin nomograms for treatment decisions
3. Phototherapy is highly effective if started early
4. Exchange transfusion is lifesaving but requires specialized care

CHAPTER 29:
Neonatal Sepsis

Overview

Neonatal sepsis is a systemic infection occurring in infants less than 28 days old, characterized by nonspecific signs and rapid deterioration. Early recognition and initiation of broad-spectrum antibiotics and supportive care are critical to reduce morbidity and mortality, especially in rural settings.

Red Flags – "Don't Miss" Features

1. Temperature instability (fever or hypothermia)
2. Poor feeding or vomiting
3. Respiratory distress, apnea, or grunting
4. Lethargy, irritability, or seizures
5. Hypotension or poor perfusion
6. Abdominal distension or jaundice

Initial Assessment in the Rural ER

1. Assess airway, breathing, and circulation promptly
2. Obtain full set of vital signs including temperature
3. Detailed history including maternal infections, delivery complications, and prenatal care
4. Physical exam for signs of infection, organ dysfunction, and hydration status

Stabilization Protocol

1. Establish IV or IO access immediately
2. Begin oxygen supplementation if hypoxic
3. Administer isotonic fluid bolus (20 mL/kg) if signs of shock
4. Start empiric broad-spectrum antibiotics urgently:

5. Ampicillin + Gentamicin or Cefotaxime
6. Monitor blood glucose and treat hypoglycemia
7. Manage seizures or respiratory support as needed

Investigations

1. CBC with differential
2. Blood culture before antibiotics if possible
3. Urinalysis and urine culture via catheterization
4. Lumbar puncture if stable and no contraindications
5. Chest x-ray if respiratory symptoms present

Differential Diagnosis

1. Bacterial sepsis
2. Viral infections (e.g., HSV, enterovirus)
3. Metabolic disorders
4. Congenital anomalies
5. Respiratory distress syndrome

Management in the Rural Setting

1. Start antibiotics promptly after cultures
2. Maintain supportive care with fluids, oxygen, and temperature control
3. Monitor closely for deterioration or response to therapy
4. Prepare for urgent transfer to tertiary care if unstable or complications present
5. Collaborate with pediatric specialists remotely if possible

Disposition and Transfer Criteria

1. **Urgent transfer** for all neonates with suspected sepsis
2. Transfer if respiratory failure, shock, or organ dysfunction
3. Admit locally only if stable and with close monitoring capabilities

Parental Communication & Reassurance

1. Explain the severity and need for urgent treatment
2. Educate on signs of worsening and importance of follow-up
3. Provide clear information about the treatment plan and transfer
4. Offer emotional support and answer questions patiently

Documentation Essentials

1. Precise description of symptoms and onset
2. Vital signs and physical exam findings
3. Antibiotics administered and timing
4. Communication with family and transfer details
5. Laboratory and imaging results

Practical Pearls for Rural Docs

1. Neonates can deteriorate rapidly—early recognition is vital
2. Blood cultures should be taken before antibiotics but do not delay treatment
3. Ampicillin plus gentamicin remains first-line empiric therapy
4. Use weight-based dosing and double-check calculations

CHAPTER 30:
Non-Accidental Trauma / Safeguarding Concerns

Overview

Non-Accidental Trauma (NAT) refers to intentional injury inflicted on a child, often called child abuse. Early recognition and safeguarding are critical to prevent further harm. Rural providers must be vigilant for subtle signs and ensure timely reporting and protection.

Red Flags – "Don't Miss" Features

1. Inconsistent or vague history of injury
2. Delayed presentation or recurrent injuries
3. Injuries in non-ambulatory children (bruises, fractures)
4. Multiple fractures at different healing stages
5. Patterned bruises or burns
6. Injuries inconsistent with developmental abilities
7. Behavioral signs: fearful, withdrawn, or aggressive

Initial Assessment in the Rural ER

1. Ensure ABCs and stabilize as needed
2. Full head-to-toe examination documenting all injuries
3. Photographic documentation if possible
4. Assess neuro status and pain level
5. Interview child and caregivers separately if safe and appropriate

Stabilization Protocol

1. Treat injuries as per standard protocols (fractures, head trauma, burns)
2. Manage pain adequately

3. Monitor for signs of neglect or malnutrition
4. Prepare for transfer to tertiary center if severe injuries or concerns

Investigations

1. Skeletal survey to detect occult fractures
2. Head CT for suspected intracranial injury
3. Laboratory tests to rule out bleeding disorders
4. Screening for sexual abuse if indicated
5. Consult child protection teams for guidance

Differential Diagnosis

1. Accidental trauma with clear history
2. Medical conditions causing bruising (e.g., bleeding disorders)
3. Osteogenesis imperfecta or metabolic bone disease
4. Cultural practices (coining, cupping)
5. Dermatoses mimicking injury

Management in the Rural Setting

1. Report all suspected cases promptly to child protection services as mandated by law
2. Maintain a non-judgmental approach with caregivers
3. Coordinate with multidisciplinary teams (social work, pediatrics, law enforcement)
4. Ensure child safety prior to discharge or transfer
5. Provide psychological support where possible

Disposition and Transfer Criteria

Transfer if:

1. Severe injuries requiring specialist care
2. Concerns for ongoing risk or unsafe home environment

3. Need for detailed investigations or legal evaluation
4. Admit or observe locally if safe and stable with social support

Parental Communication & Reassurance

1. Approach conversations with sensitivity and care
2. Avoid accusations during initial assessment
3. Explain the need for safeguarding to protect the child
4. Provide resources and support for families when appropriate

Documentation Essentials

1. Detailed, objective recording of injuries with measurements
2. Photographs if permitted
3. Statements from child and caregivers verbatim if possible
4. Notes on reporting and referrals made
5. Legal and ethical considerations documented

Practical Pearls for Rural Docs

1. Trust your clinical suspicion; early reporting saves lives
2. Be aware of local laws on mandatory reporting
3. Multidisciplinary approach is essential for best outcomes
4. Document thoroughly and objectively

CHAPTER 31:
Otitis Media / Mastoiditis

Overview

Acute otitis media (AOM) is a common bacterial infection of the middle ear, mostly affecting infants and young children. Mastoiditis is a serious complication involving infection of the mastoid air cells. Early diagnosis and management are important to prevent hearing loss and intracranial complications.

Red Flags – "Don't Miss" Features

1. Persistent high fever (>39°C) despite antibiotics
2. Severe ear pain and swelling behind the ear
3. Protruding ear or erythema over mastoid area
4. Postauricular tenderness and fluctuance
5. Hearing loss or speech delay
6. Signs of intracranial extension: headache, vomiting, altered consciousness

Initial Assessment in the Rural ER

1. Vital signs including temperature
2. Ear examination with otoscope: bulging, erythematous tympanic membrane
3. Look for mastoid swelling, erythema, tenderness
4. Assess for signs of systemic illness or neurologic changes
5. Obtain history of fever duration, ear discharge, and prior antibiotic use

Stabilization Protocol

1. Pain control with acetaminophen or ibuprofen
2. Initiate empiric oral antibiotics for AOM (e.g., Amoxicillin 80–90 mg/kg/day divided BID)
3. IV antibiotics if mastoiditis suspected or toxic appearance
4. Admit if mastoiditis suspected for IV antibiotics and monitoring
5. Supportive care: hydration, fever control

Investigations

1. Consider CBC and inflammatory markers if severe or mastoiditis suspected
2. Culture of ear discharge if present
3. Imaging (CT or MRI) if mastoiditis suspected to evaluate extent
4. Audiology referral if recurrent or complicated AOM

Differential Diagnosis

1. Viral upper respiratory infection with ear pain
2. Foreign body in ear canal
3. Otitis externa
4. Chronic suppurative otitis media
5. Mastoiditis and intracranial complications

Management in the Rural Setting

1. Start oral antibiotics promptly for uncomplicated AOM
2. Early referral for imaging and specialist care if mastoiditis suspected
3. Monitor for response to therapy; admit if worsening or systemic signs
4. Educate caregivers on medication adherence and signs of complications

Disposition and Transfer Criteria

1. **Discharge** if mild AOM with reliable follow-up and no systemic signs
2. **Admit locally or transfer** if mastoiditis suspected or patient toxic
3. Urgent transfer if signs of intracranial involvement or airway compromise
4. Early specialist consultation for complicated cases

Parental Communication & Reassurance

1. Explain typical course of AOM and importance of antibiotics
2. Reassure about usually good prognosis with treatment
3. Advise on when to return (persistent fever, worsening ear pain, swelling)
4. Educate on prevention measures (avoid smoke exposure, hand hygiene)

Documentation Essentials

1. Ear exam findings including tympanic membrane appearance
2. Vital signs and systemic assessment
3. Antibiotics prescribed and dosing
4. Follow-up and transfer plans
5. Communication with parents/caregivers

Practical Pearls for Rural Docs

1. Amoxicillin remains first-line for uncomplicated AOM
2. Mastoiditis requires prompt IV antibiotics and imaging
3. Watch for signs of intracranial spread (headache, neurological symptoms)
4. Pain control improves patient comfort and compliance

CHAPTER 32:
Pediatric Airway Management & Rapid Sequence Intubation (RSI)

Overview

Airway management in pediatric emergencies is vital to ensure oxygenation and ventilation. Rapid Sequence Intubation (RSI) is a controlled method of securing the airway while minimizing risks. Knowledge of pediatric anatomy, drug dosing, and equipment is crucial for safe and effective intubation in rural settings.

Red Flags – "Don't Miss" Features

1. Airway obstruction signs: stridor, retractions, cyanosis
2. Respiratory failure or apnea
3. Altered level of consciousness with compromised airway protection
4. Need for mechanical ventilation or airway protection during procedures
5. Failed initial airway maneuvers or bag-mask ventilation

Initial Assessment in the Rural ER

1. Assess airway patency, breathing adequacy, and circulation
2. Prepare all necessary equipment (pediatric sizes of blades, tubes, suction)
3. Review patient weight for drug dosing and equipment sizing
4. Assign roles for airway management team
5. Ensure monitoring devices are functional (pulse oximetry, capnography)

Stabilization Protocol

1. Pre-oxygenate with 100% oxygen using bag-mask or non-rebreather mask
2. Prepare RSI medications: sedative (e.g., ketamine, etomidate) and paralytic (e.g., rocuronium, succinylcholine)
3. Perform rapid sequence intubation following protocol
4. Confirm tube placement with capnography and auscultation
5. Secure endotracheal tube and initiate ventilation

Investigations

1. Not usually required pre-intubation but obtain ABGs post-intubation
2. Continuous pulse oximetry and end-tidal CO2 monitoring
3. Chest x-ray post-intubation to confirm tube position

Differential Diagnosis

1. Upper airway obstruction (croup, foreign body)
2. Lower airway disease (asthma, bronchiolitis)
3. Central nervous system depression or trauma
4. Respiratory muscle fatigue or neuromuscular disorders

Management in the Rural Setting

1. Prepare airway equipment and medications ahead of time
2. Use appropriate weight-based dosing for medications
3. Anticipate complications and have backup airway devices ready
4. Use checklists and team communication protocols
5. Plan for transfer post-intubation to higher-level care

Disposition and Transfer Criteria

1. Transfer after intubation for all patients needing advanced respiratory support
2. Monitor vital signs and ventilator settings during transport
3. Communicate airway details to receiving team

Parental Communication & Reassurance

1. Explain the need for airway support and intubation
2. Provide updates on procedure and patient status
3. Offer emotional support and answer questions clearly

Documentation Essentials

1. Time and indications for intubation
2. Drugs used with doses and times
3. Number of attempts and success
4. Confirmation methods and tube size
5. Ventilation settings and patient response

Practical Pearls for Rural Docs

1. Pediatric airway anatomy differs—smaller, more anterior, and easily obstructed
2. Use Broselow tape for quick weight and dose calculations
3. Always have suction ready and backup airway devices
4. Confirm tube placement with end-tidal CO_2 and chest auscultation

CHAPTER 33:
Pediatric Trauma Assessment (ATLS Adaptation)

Overview

Pediatric trauma assessment requires a systematic approach adapted from Advanced Trauma Life Support (ATLS) principles. Children have unique anatomical and physiological differences that influence injury patterns and resuscitation priorities. Early identification of life-threatening injuries and stabilization are critical in rural emergency care.

Red Flags – "Don't Miss" Features

1. Altered level of consciousness or GCS <15
2. Respiratory distress or apnea
3. Signs of shock or poor perfusion
4. Open fractures or suspected long bone fractures
5. Abdominal tenderness or distension
6. Signs of head or spinal injury (neck pain, paralysis)
7. Deformities, swelling, or bleeding

Initial Assessment in the Rural ER

1. Follow ABCDE approach:
2. Airway with cervical spine protection
3. Breathing: assess work of breathing, breath sounds, chest movement
4. Circulation: check pulses, capillary refill, hemorrhage control
5. Disability: neurological status (AVPU/GCS), pupil assessment
6. Exposure: complete head-to-toe exam, temperature control
7. Use pediatric-specific assessment tools and weight-based calculations
8. Obtain history of injury mechanism and timing

Stabilization Protocol

1. Secure airway, prepare for advanced airway if needed
2. Provide supplemental oxygen and assist ventilation if required
3. Control external bleeding and establish IV/IO access
4. Administer isotonic fluid boluses (20 mL/kg) for shock
5. Monitor vital signs continuously
6. Immobilize suspected fractures and spine

Investigations

1. Rapid bedside glucose and oxygen saturation
2. CBC, blood type and crossmatch if significant bleeding
3. Portable chest and pelvis x-rays
4. Focused assessment with sonography for trauma (FAST) if available
5. CT imaging if indicated and available

Differential Diagnosis

1. Traumatic brain injury (concussion, intracranial hemorrhage)
2. Thoracic injuries (pneumothorax, hemothorax)
3. Abdominal trauma (splenic or liver injury)
4. Long bone fractures
5. Spinal cord injury
6. Soft tissue injuries

Management in the Rural Setting

1. Prioritize airway and breathing interventions
2. Use fluid resuscitation judiciously, avoiding overload
3. Control bleeding and prevent hypothermia
4. Arrange rapid transfer to trauma center if indicated
5. Provide analgesia carefully
6. Communicate clearly with receiving team

Disposition and Transfer Criteria

Transfer urgently if:

1. Airway compromise or inability to protect airway
2. Respiratory failure or persistent hypoxia
3. Signs of shock unresponsive to fluids
4. Head injury with decreased consciousness
5. Multiple or unstable fractures
6. Need for surgical intervention or ICU care

Parental Communication & Reassurance

1. Explain the trauma assessment steps and findings
2. Provide updates on interventions and transfer plans
3. Offer emotional support and clear communication
4. Prepare family for transfer and possible outcomes

Documentation Essentials

1. Time and mechanism of injury
2. ABCDE findings and vital signs
3. Interventions and fluid volumes administered
4. Imaging and lab results
5. Communication with family and transfer documentation

Practical Pearls for Rural Docs

1. Children compensate well until sudden decompensation—monitor closely
2. Maintain cervical spine precautions until cleared
3. Use Broselow tape or weight-based formulas for meds and equipment
4. Early communication with trauma referral center improves outcomes

CHAPTER 34:
Peritonsillar & Retropharyngeal Abscess

Overview

Peritonsillar and retropharyngeal abscesses are deep neck space infections often complicating tonsillitis or pharyngitis. They can cause airway obstruction, severe pain, and systemic toxicity. Prompt diagnosis and airway assessment are vital in rural emergency care.

Red Flags – "Don't Miss" Features

1. Severe sore throat with unilateral swelling or trismus
2. Muffled "hot potato" voice
3. Neck stiffness and torticollis (retropharyngeal abscess)
4. Drooling and difficulty swallowing
5. Fever and toxic appearance
6. Respiratory distress or stridor

Initial Assessment in the Rural ER

1. Assess airway patency and respiratory effort
2. Vital signs and oxygen saturation
3. Examine oropharynx carefully (avoid agitation)
4. Neck exam for swelling, tenderness, or stiffness
5. Obtain history of symptom progression and prior infections

Stabilization Protocol

1. Secure airway if compromised
2. Oxygen therapy if hypoxic
3. IV fluids for hydration and sepsis
4. Empiric IV antibiotics targeting common pathogens (see management)
5. Analgesia and fever control

Investigations

1. CBC, blood cultures if febrile or toxic
2. Imaging (contrast-enhanced CT neck) to confirm abscess and extent
3. Consider lateral neck x-ray if CT unavailable but less sensitive
4. Throat swab cultures if safe

Differential Diagnosis

1. Peritonsillar cellulitis
2. Retropharyngeal cellulitis
3. Infectious mononucleosis
4. Epiglottitis
5. Deep neck space tumors

Management in the Rural Setting

1. Early antibiotic therapy targeting Streptococcus, Staphylococcus, anaerobes
2. Consider corticosteroids to reduce swelling
3. Consult ENT for possible drainage (needle aspiration or incision)
4. Transfer urgently if airway compromise or extensive infection
5. Supportive care: fluids, analgesics

Disposition and Transfer Criteria

1. **Urgent transfer** if airway obstruction or respiratory distress
2. Transfer for imaging or surgical drainage if not available locally
3. Admit locally if mild and improving, with close monitoring and ENT follow-up

Parental Communication & Reassurance

1. Explain seriousness of deep neck infections
2. Discuss need for hospital admission or transfer
3. Reassure regarding treatment plan and follow-up

Documentation Essentials

1. Airway status and respiratory assessment
2. Imaging and lab results
3. Antibiotics administered and response
4. Consultations and transfer details

Practical Pearls for Rural Docs

1. Do not attempt throat exam if airway compromise suspected
2. Early ENT consultation reduces complications
3. Steroids may speed recovery but should not delay antibiotics
4. Always consider deep neck infections in severe sore throat with swelling

CHAPTER 35:
Pneumonia – Bacterial and Viral

Overview

Pneumonia is a common cause of fever and respiratory distress in children. It can be bacterial or viral, with overlapping presentations. Bacterial pneumonia is often more abrupt with high fever and localized findings, while viral pneumonia presents more gradually with diffuse symptoms. Prompt recognition and appropriate antibiotic use are essential in rural settings.

Red Flags – "Don't Miss" Features

1. Toxic appearance, lethargy, or poor perfusion
2. Severe respiratory distress (nasal flaring, retractions, grunting)
3. Oxygen saturation <90% on room air
4. Chest pain or abdominal pain (referred from lower lobe involvement)
5. Signs of sepsis (tachycardia, delayed cap refill, hypotension)
6. Age <6 months or underlying comorbidities (CHD, immunodeficiency)

Initial Assessment in the Rural ER

1. Assess airway, breathing, and circulation
2. Vital signs including SpO2 and temperature
3. Full respiratory exam: work of breathing, breath sounds, crackles, dullness
4. Assess hydration status and ability to feed/drink
5. Brief history: cough, fever, duration, sick contacts, vaccinations

Stabilization Protocol

1. Provide oxygen to maintain SpO2 >92%
2. IV or oral fluids depending on hydration status
3. Antipyretics for comfort
4. Initiate empiric antibiotics if bacterial pneumonia suspected:
5. <5 years: Amoxicillin 80–90 mg/kg/day divided BID (PO)
6. ≥5 years or atypical signs: add macrolide (Azithromycin 10 mg/kg day 1, then 5 mg/kg days 2–5)
7. Unable to tolerate PO or toxic: Ceftriaxone 50–75 mg/kg IV/IM daily

Investigations

1. CBC, blood cultures (if febrile or toxic-appearing)
2. Chest x-ray (not required for all; helpful if hypoxia, failed treatment, or uncertain diagnosis)
3. CRP or procalcitonin (if available) may help distinguish viral vs bacterial
4. Nasopharyngeal swab for viral PCR during respiratory season (optional)

Differential Diagnosis

1. Bacterial pneumonia (Strep pneumoniae, H. influenzae, S. aureus)
2. Viral pneumonia (RSV, influenza, adenovirus, parainfluenza)
3. Bronchiolitis (esp. in infants <1 year)
4. Asthma exacerbation
5. Foreign body aspiration
6. Tuberculosis (rare in Canada, consider travel or TB exposure)

Management in the Rural Setting

1. Treat based on severity: oral antibiotics for mild cases; IV antibiotics for moderate to severe or vomiting children
2. Provide oxygen and supportive care (fluids, fever control)
3. Monitor closely for deterioration (increased WOB, poor feeding, cyanosis)
4. Educate caregivers on red flags and follow-up needs

Disposition and Transfer Criteria

Discharge if:

1. Mild pneumonia, tolerating fluids, SpO2 >92%, normal RR for age, no comorbidities
2. **Observe** in ED or short-stay if uncertain or borderline hypoxic

Transfer if:

1. SpO2 <90% or requiring >2L/min oxygen
2. Moderate–severe respiratory distress or dehydration
3. Concern for sepsis, effusion/empyema, or failed oral therapy

Parental Communication & Reassurance

1. Explain likely cause (bacterial vs viral) and rationale for antibiotics
2. Review medication dosing and completion of course
3. Teach signs of worsening (e.g., fast breathing, poor feeding, color change)
4. Ensure follow-up within 24–48 hours, sooner if deteriorating

Documentation Essentials

1. Vital signs and respiratory findings
2. CXR findings (if done) and rationale for antibiotics or not
3. Medications given and prescriptions provided
4. Disposition decision and caregiver instructions

Practical Pearls for Rural Docs

1. Amoxicillin remains first-line for most bacterial pneumonia
2. Don't overuse chest x-ray—clinical diagnosis is often sufficient
3. Young infants can decompensate quickly—monitor and reassess often
4. Pneumonia can mimic abdominal pain or asthma—consider broad differential

CHAPTER 36:
Pyloric Stenosis

Overview

Hypertrophic pyloric stenosis is a condition causing gastric outlet obstruction in infants, typically presenting at 3–6 weeks of age. It results from hypertrophy of the pyloric muscle, leading to projectile non-bilious vomiting, dehydration, and weight loss. Early diagnosis and surgical referral are key.

Red Flags – "Don't Miss" Features

1. Projectile non-bilious vomiting
2. Palpable "olive" mass in the right upper quadrant
3. Dehydration signs: dry mucous membranes, lethargy
4. Weight loss or failure to thrive
5. Visible peristalsis across the abdomen

Initial Assessment in the Rural ER

1. Assess hydration and vital signs
2. Evaluate vomiting characteristics and feeding tolerance
3. Perform abdominal exam for palpable mass and peristalsis
4. Obtain history of symptom duration and weight changes

Stabilization Protocol

1. Correct dehydration with IV fluids, monitor electrolytes
2. Avoid oral feeds until surgical evaluation
3. Prepare for surgical consultation and transfer
4. Monitor urine output and clinical status

Investigations

1. Ultrasound abdomen to confirm hypertrophied pylorus
2. Electrolytes and blood gas to assess metabolic alkalosis
3. CBC to evaluate for infection or anemia

Differential Diagnosis

1. Gastroesophageal reflux
2. Gastroenteritis
3. Malrotation with obstruction
4. Other causes of vomiting and failure to thrive

Management in the Rural Setting

1. Initiate fluid resuscitation and correct electrolyte imbalances
2. Avoid oral intake until definitive diagnosis and surgery
3. Arrange urgent transfer to pediatric surgery center
4. Provide supportive care and analgesia

Disposition and Transfer Criteria

1. Urgent transfer for all suspected cases
2. Ensure stabilization prior to transfer
3. Monitor for worsening dehydration or electrolyte imbalance

Parental Communication & Reassurance

1. Explain the nature of the condition and need for surgery
2. Reassure about the generally good surgical outcomes
3. Provide clear instructions on feeding and hydration before transfer

Documentation Essentials

1. Vomiting characteristics and abdominal exam findings
2. Fluid resuscitation details
3. Imaging and lab results
4. Communication with family and receiving team

Practical Pearls for Rural Docs

1. Classic presentation is projectile non-bilious vomiting at 3–6 weeks
2. Palpable "olive" is pathognomonic but may be subtle
3. Metabolic alkalosis is common—correct before surgery
4. Early surgical referral improves outcomes

CHAPTER 37:
Rashes – Emergency vs Benign

Overview

Rashes are a common presentation in children and can range from benign viral exanthems to life-threatening conditions. In the rural ER setting, rapid assessment is essential to identify serious causes and differentiate them from self-limited illnesses. A focused history and exam can guide urgency and need for transfer.

Red Flags – "Don't Miss" Features

1. Non-blanching petechiae or purpura (e.g., meningococcemia)
2. Rapidly spreading erythema with systemic illness (e.g., toxic shock, necrotizing fasciitis)
3. Mucosal involvement (e.g., Stevens-Johnson syndrome, Kawasaki disease)
4. Bullous lesions or epidermal detachment (e.g., SJS/TEN, staphylococcal scalded skin syndrome)
5. Associated hypotension, altered mental status, or fever >39°C
6. Pain out of proportion to appearance
7. Recent medication use or known allergy

Initial Assessment in the Rural ER

1. Assess vital signs and overall appearance
2. Determine timing and progression of rash
3. Ask about recent infections, medications, allergies, or travel
4. Examine full skin surface and mucous membranes
5. Look for blanching, pattern (macular, vesicular, petechial), and associated symptoms

Stabilization Protocol

1. Stabilize ABCs if systemic illness present
2. Administer IV fluids for hypotension
3. Empiric antibiotics if meningococcemia or sepsis suspected
4. Antihistamines or corticosteroids if allergic reaction or urticaria
5. Analgesia and skin care as needed
6. Protect skin if epidermal loss (e.g., SJS/TEN)

Investigations

1. CBC, CRP, blood cultures if febrile or toxic-appearing
2. Throat swab or rapid strep test if pharyngitis suspected
3. Skin swab for bacterial culture if oozing lesions
4. Consider LP if signs of meningitis with petechial rash
5. CXR if respiratory symptoms present

Differential Diagnosis

1. Benign viral exanthems (roseola, measles, rubella, fifth disease)
2. Hand-Foot-Mouth Disease (coxsackievirus)
3. Allergic urticaria or drug eruption
4. Bacterial: cellulitis, impetigo, scarlet fever
5. Meningococcemia
6. Kawasaki disease
7. Toxic shock syndrome
8. Stevens-Johnson syndrome / Toxic epidermal necrolysis

Management in the Rural Setting

1. Reassure and discharge if afebrile and well-appearing with benign viral rash
2. Treat bacterial skin infections with appropriate antibiotics
3. Start IV antibiotics immediately if purpura or systemic illness present
4. Administer antipyretics and hydration support

5. Arrange urgent transfer for suspected SJS/TEN, meningococcemia, or Kawasaki disease
6. Document rash appearance and progression clearly

Disposition and Transfer Criteria

1. Transfer urgently if signs of systemic illness, purpura, bullae, or mucosal involvement
2. Stable viral rashes can be discharged with outpatient follow-up
3. Refer for dermatology or infectious disease input if uncertain diagnosis and not improving

Parental Communication & Reassurance

1. Explain likely benign vs concerning features of rash
2. Give clear return precautions (fever, behavioral change, rash spread)
3. Provide instructions for hydration, fever control, and skin care
4. Discuss allergy history and medication risks if reaction suspected

Documentation Essentials

1. Complete rash description: type, distribution, blanching, mucosal involvement
2. Vital signs and systemic symptoms
3. Recent illness, exposures, or medications
4. Treatments given and disposition plan
5. Parental counselling and return instructions

Practical Pearls for Rural Docs

1. Blanching vs non-blanching is a critical initial distinction
2. Petechiae and purpura always warrant serious consideration
3. Mucosal and eye involvement point to systemic illness
4. Use photos (with consent) for documentation if helpful

5. When in doubt, consult pediatrics or dermatology early

CHAPTER 38:
Seizures & Status Epilepticus

Overview

Seizures are a common pediatric emergency and may be due to febrile illness, epilepsy, CNS infections, metabolic disturbances, trauma, or toxins. Status epilepticus is defined as continuous seizure activity >5 minutes or recurrent seizures without return to baseline consciousness between events.

Red Flags – "Don't Miss" Features

1. Seizure lasting >5 minutes
2. Focal features (e.g., gaze deviation, hemiparesis)
3. Prolonged postictal state or failure to regain consciousness
4. Fever, neck stiffness, bulging fontanelle (meningitis signs)
5. Signs of trauma or non-accidental injury
6. Hypoxia, cyanosis, hypotension

Initial Assessment in the Rural ER

1. ABCs and Pediatric Triangle (Appearance, Work of Breathing, Circulation)
2. Vital signs (age-appropriate HR, RR, BP, O2 Sat)
3. Blood glucose (fingerstick)
4. Neurological status: GCS, focal deficits, postictal phase
5. History: duration, focality, recent illness, trauma, medications, past history of seizures

Stabilization Protocol

1. **Airway**: Position airway, suction, O2, airway adjuncts if needed
2. **Breathing**: Ensure oxygenation; bag-valve-mask if apneic

3. **Circulation**: Establish IV or IO access; monitor HR, BP
4. **Disability**: Check glucose; treat hypoglycemia if present

Drugs:

1. First line: Lorazepam IV 0.1 mg/kg (max 4 mg) or Midazolam IM/intranasal/buccal 0.2 mg/kg
2. Second line: Fosphenytoin 20 mg PE/kg IV or Phenobarbital
3. Consider intubation and RSI if refractory seizures

Investigations

1. Fingerstick glucose (immediate)
2. CBC, electrolytes, calcium, magnesium, urea, creatinine
3. Antiepileptic drug levels (if known seizure disorder)
4. Blood cultures if febrile
5. CT head (if trauma, focal findings, concern for bleed)
6. Lumbar puncture if concern for meningitis/encephalitis (after imaging if needed)

Differential Diagnosis

1. Febrile seizure
2. Epilepsy (known or new onset)
3. CNS infection (meningitis, encephalitis)
4. Head trauma / intracranial hemorrhage
5. Metabolic (hypoglycemia, hyponatremia)
6. Toxin ingestion / drug overdose
7. Non-epileptic spells (e.g., breath-holding, syncope, pseudo-seizure)

Management in the Rural Setting

1. ABC management
2. Weight-based medication dosing (always calculate)
3. Monitor vitals and seizure activity continuously

4. Keep resuscitation drugs ready
5. Initiate antiepileptic loading if benzodiazepines fail

Disposition and Transfer Criteria

1. Admit locally if seizures resolve, patient is stable, and no red flags

Urgent transfer if:

1. Refractory status epilepticus
2. Concerns for CNS infection or structural brain lesion
3. Needs EEG or neuroimaging not available locally
4. Ensure IV access and stabilize prior to transfer
5. Notify receiving pediatric or PICU team early

Parental Communication & Reassurance

1. Explain common causes of seizures and warning signs
2. Clarify febrile vs afebrile seizures
3. Provide return precautions if discharged
4. Discuss medication plan and follow-up if seizure disorder suspected

Documentation Essentials

1. Time of seizure onset and resolution
2. All interventions and drug doses
3. Neurological exam and vital signs pre- and post-event
4. Parental discussions and transfer notes if applicable

Practical Pearls for Rural Docs

1. Always check glucose early in any seizure
2. Buccal/intranasal midazolam is safe and fast if IV not available
3. Have a Broselow tape or pediatric dosing sheet handy
4. Use weight-based dosing strictly; avoid under/overdosing

CHAPTER 39:
Sepsis & Fever Without Source (Neonates, Infants)

Overview

Sepsis and fever without source in neonates and young infants present a diagnostic challenge. These patients are at high risk for serious bacterial infections and rapid deterioration. Prompt recognition, early empiric antibiotic therapy, and careful monitoring are essential in rural settings where specialized pediatric resources may be limited.

Red Flags – "Don't Miss" Features

1. Temperature ≥38°C (100.4°F) in neonates <28 days
2. Poor feeding, lethargy, irritability
3. Respiratory distress or apnea
4. Hypotension or poor perfusion
5. Altered mental status or seizures
6. Persistent high fever without localizing signs

Initial Assessment in the Rural ER

1. ABCs: airway patency, breathing adequacy, circulation
2. Obtain full vital signs including temperature, HR, RR, BP, and O2 saturation
3. Detailed history including perinatal factors, maternal infections, immunizations
4. Focused physical exam to exclude focal infections (otitis, pneumonia, UTI, meningitis)
5. Assess hydration and neurological status

Stabilization Protocol

1. Establish IV or IO access promptly
2. Begin oxygen therapy if hypoxic
3. Administer isotonic fluid bolus 20 mL/kg if signs of shock
4. Initiate empiric broad-spectrum antibiotics without delay:
5. Neonates (<28 days): Ampicillin + Gentamicin (or Cefotaxime if meningitis suspected)
6. Infants (>28 days to 3 months): Ceftriaxone or Cefotaxime + Vancomycin (if MRSA suspected)
7. Monitor glucose and treat hypoglycemia if present
8. Manage seizures or respiratory distress as needed

Investigations

1. CBC with differential
2. Blood culture prior to antibiotics
3. Urinalysis and urine culture (catheterized specimen preferred)
4. Lumbar puncture if no contraindications and stable
5. Chest x-ray if respiratory symptoms
6. Viral testing if available (RSV, influenza)

Differential Diagnosis

1. Serious bacterial infection (sepsis, meningitis, UTI, pneumonia)
2. Viral infections (RSV, influenza, enterovirus)
3. Metabolic causes (hypoglycemia, inborn errors)
4. Congenital heart disease with fever
5. Non-infectious causes of fever

Management in the Rural Setting

1. Start antibiotics as soon as IV/IO access obtained
2. Maintain supportive care and fluid resuscitation
3. Monitor closely for deterioration or response to treatment

4. Early consultation with pediatric or infectious disease specialists if available
5. Arrange urgent transfer to tertiary care if unstable or diagnosis uncertain

Disposition and Transfer Criteria

1. **Urgent transfer** for all neonates (<28 days) with fever
2. Transfer for any infant with signs of shock or instability
3. Stable infants >28 days may be observed locally with close monitoring if no red flags
4. Transfer if lumbar puncture or imaging needed and unavailable locally

Parental Communication & Reassurance

1. Explain potential severity and need for prompt treatment
2. Educate on signs of worsening and importance of follow-up
3. Provide clear instructions about the plan, transfer, and treatment
4. Reassure that many infants recover fully with early care

Documentation Essentials

1. Precise temperature and timing of fever
2. Vital signs and physical exam findings
3. Antibiotics given (dose, time)
4. Communication with parents and transfer team
5. Results of investigations as they return

Practical Pearls for Rural Docs

1. Fever in neonates is a medical emergency until proven otherwise
2. Blood cultures should be obtained before antibiotics if possible but don't delay therapy

3. LP timing depends on stability—never delay antibiotics for LP if unstable
4. Use weight-based dosing and double-check with dosing tools

CHAPTER 40:
Testicular Torsion / Ovarian Torsion

Overview

Testicular and ovarian torsion are surgical emergencies caused by twisting of the spermatic cord or ovarian pedicle, leading to ischemia. Rapid diagnosis and urgent intervention are vital to preserve gonadal function.

Red Flags – "Don't Miss" Features

1. Sudden onset severe scrotal or lower abdominal pain
2. Swelling and erythema of scrotum or lower abdomen
3. Nausea and vomiting
4. Absent cremasteric reflex (testicular torsion)
5. High-riding or horizontally oriented testis

Initial Assessment in the Rural ER

1. Assess ABCs and vital signs
2. Perform careful genitourinary and abdominal exam
3. Check for swelling, tenderness, erythema
4. Assess for signs of systemic illness or sepsis
5. Obtain history of symptom onset and progression

Stabilization Protocol

1. Provide analgesia promptly
2. Maintain hydration and monitor vital signs
3. Prepare for urgent transfer to surgical center
4. Avoid delays in diagnosis and treatment

Investigations

1. Doppler ultrasound to assess blood flow (if available)
2. Urinalysis to exclude infection
3. Laboratory tests if systemic illness suspected

Differential Diagnosis

1. Epididymitis or orchitis
2. Torsion of testicular appendage
3. Incarcerated hernia
4. Ovarian cyst or tumor
5. Trauma

Management in the Rural Setting

1. Prioritize rapid recognition and analgesia
2. Avoid delays; arrange urgent transfer for surgical intervention
3. Educate caregivers about urgency and treatment steps
4. Monitor patient closely during transfer

Disposition and Transfer Criteria

1. Immediate transfer for all suspected cases
2. Stabilize and manage pain before transport
3. Communicate urgency to receiving center

Parental Communication & Reassurance

1. Explain the emergency nature and need for urgent surgery
2. Reassure about surgical outcomes with early treatment
3. Provide clear instructions on symptoms and follow-up

Documentation Essentials

1. Detailed genitourinary exam findings
2. Pain assessment and analgesia given
3. Imaging and lab results
4. Transfer communication and plans

Practical Pearls for Rural Docs

1. Time is testicle/ovary—early surgery saves function
2. Absent cremasteric reflex is a key sign for testicular torsion
3. Ultrasound is helpful but should not delay transfer
4. Educate families on warning signs of torsion

CHAPTER 41:
Tonsillitis & Pharyngitis

Overview

Tonsillitis and pharyngitis are common infections of the oropharynx in children, mostly viral but sometimes bacterial (notably Group A Streptococcus). They cause sore throat, fever, and difficulty swallowing. Prompt diagnosis is important to prevent complications like rheumatic fever and abscess formation.

Red Flags – "Don't Miss" Features

1. Severe sore throat with drooling or inability to swallow
2. Trismus (difficulty opening mouth)
3. Signs of airway obstruction (stridor, muffled voice)
4. High fever >39°C persisting beyond 48 hours
5. Cervical lymphadenopathy with swelling or tenderness
6. Presence of rash or petechiae

Initial Assessment in the Rural ER

1. Assess airway patency and breathing
2. Vital signs including temperature and hydration status
3. Inspect oropharynx for erythema, exudate, swelling
4. Palpate cervical lymph nodes
5. History of exposure to streptococcal infections or recurrent sore throats

Stabilization Protocol

1. Support airway and hydration
2. Analgesia with acetaminophen or ibuprofen
3. Encourage oral fluids if tolerated

4. Begin empiric antibiotics if bacterial tonsillitis suspected (see management)

Investigations

1. Rapid antigen detection test (if available) for GAS
2. Throat swab culture for bacterial confirmation
3. CBC and inflammatory markers if systemic illness suspected

Differential Diagnosis

1. Viral pharyngitis (adenovirus, EBV)
2. Bacterial tonsillitis (Group A Streptococcus)
3. Infectious mononucleosis
4. Peritonsillar abscess (if asymmetric swelling)
5. Allergic rhinitis or postnasal drip

Management in the Rural Setting

1. Oral penicillin or amoxicillin for confirmed or probable GAS
2. Symptomatic care for viral cases
3. Educate about importance of completing antibiotic course
4. Monitor for complications such as abscess or airway compromise

Disposition and Transfer Criteria

1. Discharge if mild symptoms and able to maintain hydration
2. Transfer if airway compromise, severe dehydration, or suspected abscess
3. Early ENT consultation for recurrent or complicated cases

Parental Communication & Reassurance

1. Explain viral vs bacterial causes and treatment rationale
2. Emphasize hydration and symptom control

3. Provide return instructions for worsening symptoms or airway difficulty

Documentation Essentials

1. Oropharyngeal exam findings
2. Vital signs and hydration status
3. Antibiotics prescribed and dosing
4. Parental education and disposition plan

Practical Pearls for Rural Docs

1. Most sore throats are viral and self-limited
2. Rapid tests aid diagnosis but do not replace clinical judgment
3. Avoid unnecessary antibiotics to prevent resistance
4. Watch for signs of peritonsillar abscess in persistent unilateral symptoms

CHAPTER 42:
UTI & Pyelonephritis

Overview

Urinary tract infections (UTIs) are common in children and can range from cystitis to pyelonephritis. Prompt diagnosis and treatment prevent renal scarring and complications. Young children may present with nonspecific symptoms, requiring high clinical suspicion in rural emergency settings.

Red Flags – "Don't Miss" Features

1. Fever without focus, especially in infants <2 years
2. Vomiting, poor feeding, irritability
3. Flank pain or tenderness
4. Recurrent UTIs or known urinary tract abnormalities
5. Signs of sepsis in pyelonephritis
6. Dysuria, frequency, or urgency in toilet-trained children

Initial Assessment in the Rural ER

1. Obtain vital signs and hydration status
2. Obtain thorough history including urinary symptoms and previous infections
3. Perform abdominal and genital exam for tenderness and abnormalities
4. Collect urine sample (clean catch, catheterization, or suprapubic aspiration)
5. Monitor for signs of systemic illness

Stabilization Protocol

1. Initiate IV fluids if dehydrated
2. Start empiric antibiotics based on local guidelines and age

3. Provide analgesia as needed
4. Monitor for signs of deterioration or sepsis

Investigations

1. Urinalysis and urine culture
2. CBC and blood cultures if febrile or toxic-appearing
3. Renal and bladder ultrasound for recurrent infections or atypical cases
4. Consider voiding cystourethrogram (VCUG) if indicated

Differential Diagnosis

1. Viral illness with fever
2. Gastroenteritis
3. Pyelonephritis
4. Vaginitis or balanitis
5. Constipation

Management in the Rural Setting

1. Treat with appropriate antibiotics promptly
2. Support hydration and monitor clinical response
3. Refer for imaging if recurrent or complicated infections
4. Educate caregivers on hygiene and prevention

Disposition and Transfer Criteria

1. Transfer if septic or unable to maintain hydration
2. Admit locally if mild pyelonephritis requiring IV antibiotics
3. Discharge with oral antibiotics if stable and able to tolerate fluids
4. Arrange outpatient follow-up and imaging

Parental Communication & Reassurance

1. Explain importance of completing antibiotics
2. Educate about hygiene and signs of worsening
3. Reassure on prognosis with treatment
4. Provide clear instructions on follow-up

Documentation Essentials

1. Urine collection method and results
2. Antibiotics given and response
3. Vital signs and hydration status
4. Communication and follow-up plans

Practical Pearls for Rural Docs

1. Obtain sterile urine samples for accurate diagnosis
2. Consider pyelonephritis in febrile infants without source
3. Early treatment prevents renal scarring
4. Educate families on prevention and hydration

CHAPTER 43:
Volvulus / Malrotation

Overview

Malrotation is a congenital anomaly of intestinal rotation and fixation that can lead to volvulus—twisting of the bowel causing obstruction and ischemia. It usually presents in neonates and young infants with bilious vomiting, abdominal distension, and shock. Immediate diagnosis and surgical intervention are critical.

Red Flags – "Don't Miss" Features

1. Bilious vomiting (green/yellow bile-stained)
2. Abdominal distension or tenderness
3. Signs of shock or lethargy
4. Bloody stools or abdominal tenderness
5. Failure to thrive or feeding intolerance

Initial Assessment in the Rural ER

1. Assess airway, breathing, and circulation
2. Obtain history of vomiting characteristics and onset
3. Examine abdomen for distension, tenderness, and signs of peritonitis
4. Monitor vital signs and neurological status

Stabilization Protocol

1. Establish IV access and begin fluid resuscitation
2. Correct electrolyte imbalances
3. Avoid oral feeding
4. Prepare for urgent surgical consultation and transfer
5. Monitor urine output and hemodynamic status

Investigations

1. Upper GI contrast study (gold standard for diagnosis)
2. Abdominal x-ray may show obstruction or gasless abdomen
3. CBC, electrolytes, blood gas analysis
4. Ultrasound may show whirlpool sign (if performed)

Differential Diagnosis

1. Malrotation with volvulus
2. Intestinal atresia or obstruction
3. Pyloric stenosis
4. Gastroenteritis
5. Sepsis

Management in the Rural Setting

1. Immediate fluid resuscitation and stabilization
2. Avoid delay in surgical transfer
3. Provide supportive care including pain management
4. Monitor for deterioration and signs of perforation

Disposition and Transfer Criteria

1. Urgent transfer to surgical center for all suspected cases
2. Stabilize before transport
3. Notify receiving team of clinical status and interventions

Parental Communication & Reassurance

1. Explain the seriousness and urgency of condition
2. Provide reassurance about surgical treatment and outcomes
3. Discuss need for transfer and monitoring

Documentation Essentials

1. Vomiting characteristics and abdominal exam findings
2. Fluid resuscitation details
3. Imaging and lab results
4. Communication with family and transfer team

Practical Pearls for Rural Docs

1. Bilious vomiting is a surgical emergency until proven otherwise
2. Early diagnosis prevents bowel necrosis and improves outcomes
3. Upper GI contrast study is diagnostic and guides surgery
4. Monitor closely for shock and electrolyte imbalances

CHAPTER 44:
Vomiting in Neonates (Malrotation, Pyloric Stenosis)

Overview

Vomiting in neonates can be caused by multiple conditions, with malrotation (with or without midgut volvulus) and hypertrophic pyloric stenosis being important surgical emergencies. Early recognition and prompt referral can prevent serious complications like bowel ischemia or severe dehydration.

Red Flags – "Don't Miss" Features

1. Bilious vomiting (green or yellow bile-stained)
2. Projectile non-bilious vomiting (pyloric stenosis)
3. Abdominal distension or tenderness
4. Failure to thrive or dehydration
5. Bloody stools or signs of shock
6. Abdominal mass (palpable "olive" in pyloric stenosis)

Initial Assessment in the Rural ER

1. Assess ABCs and hydration status
2. Obtain history of vomiting onset, frequency, bilious vs non-bilious
3. Examine abdomen for distension, tenderness, and masses
4. Assess feeding and urine output
5. Monitor vital signs and weight

Stabilization Protocol

1. Establish IV access and begin fluid resuscitation if dehydrated
2. Correct electrolyte imbalances as needed

3. Avoid oral feeds until surgical evaluation
4. Prepare for urgent transfer if surgical emergency suspected
5. Provide analgesia and monitor closely

Investigations

1. Abdominal ultrasound (for pyloric stenosis)
2. Upper GI contrast study (gold standard for malrotation diagnosis)
3. Electrolytes and blood gases
4. CBC to assess infection or anemia

Differential Diagnosis

1. Malrotation with midgut volvulus
2. Hypertrophic pyloric stenosis
3. Gastroesophageal reflux
4. Neonatal sepsis
5. Intestinal atresia or obstruction

Management in the Rural Setting

1. Early recognition and stabilization
2. Begin fluids and correct metabolic abnormalities
3. Avoid delay in surgical consultation and transfer
4. Provide supportive care including pain management
5. Educate caregivers about signs of worsening

Disposition and Transfer Criteria

1. **Urgent transfer** if bilious vomiting or signs of obstruction
2. Transfer if dehydration or electrolyte abnormalities present
3. Stable non-bilious vomiting neonates may be observed with close follow-up
4. Early surgical involvement for confirmed or suspected malrotation or pyloric stenosis

Parental Communication & Reassurance

1. Explain the seriousness of bilious vomiting and need for urgent care
2. Reassure about effective surgical treatments available
3. Provide clear instructions on monitoring feeding and vomiting
4. Discuss signs that require immediate return to hospital

Documentation Essentials

1. Detailed description of vomiting (color, frequency, volume)
2. Physical exam findings including abdominal exam
3. Interventions and response
4. Transfer communication and timing

Practical Pearls for Rural Docs

1. Bilious vomiting is a surgical emergency until proven otherwise
2. Palpable "olive" is classic for pyloric stenosis but may be subtle
3. Ultrasound is key diagnostic tool for pyloric stenosis
4. Prompt fluid resuscitation improves outcomes in obstruction

CHAPTER 45:
Weight-Based Drug Calculations & Broselow Tape Use

Overview

Weight-based drug calculations are essential for safe and effective pediatric emergency care. The Broselow Tape is a color-coded tool that provides rapid estimation of weight and corresponding drug dosages and equipment sizes, reducing errors and improving outcomes in critical situations.

Red Flags – "Don't Miss" Features

1. Risk of medication dosing errors due to weight estimation
2. Delays in drug administration in emergencies
3. Use of adult doses leading to overdose or underdose
4. Misinterpretation of Broselow tape due to unfamiliarity
5. Weight extremes (obesity, malnutrition) affecting accuracy

Initial Assessment in the Rural ER

1. Estimate or measure child's weight accurately if possible
2. Use Broselow Tape for quick weight estimation in emergencies
3. Confirm drug dosages with dosing charts or digital tools
4. Prepare all medications and equipment based on estimated weight
5. Involve trained staff for double-checking calculations

Stabilization Protocol

1. Administer medications using weight-based dosing per guidelines
2. Use Broselow Tape to select appropriate equipment sizes (ET tube, catheters)
3. Monitor patient closely for drug effects and side effects
4. Adjust doses as accurate weight becomes available
5. Document all doses given and calculations used

Investigations

1. Not applicable for drug dosing but confirm renal and liver function if possible in complex cases

Differential Diagnosis

1. Incorrect dosing due to wrong weight estimate
2. Overdose or underdose reactions
3. Drug toxicity

Management in the Rural Setting

1. Train staff regularly on Broselow Tape use and pediatric dosing
2. Maintain Broselow Tape and dosing charts in all emergency areas
3. Use electronic tools where available to cross-check doses
4. Emphasize teamwork and communication during drug administration
5. Report and learn from any medication errors

Disposition and Transfer Criteria

1. Transfer if adverse drug reactions occur or if advanced care needed

2. Ensure clear documentation and communication of medications given during transfer

Parental Communication & Reassurance

1. Explain the importance of precise dosing for safety
2. Reassure about monitoring and adjustments as needed
3. Discuss any medication side effects or concerns openly

Documentation Essentials

1. Weight estimation method and value used
2. Drug doses, timing, and route
3. Equipment sizes selected
4. Any adverse reactions or adjustments made
5. Communication with receiving team during transfers

Practical Pearls for Rural Docs

1. Broselow Tape significantly reduces medication errors in pediatric emergencies
2. Always double-check weight estimates and dosages
3. Be aware of limitations in children with atypical body habitus
4. Maintain familiarity with drug dosing protocols and emergency equipment sizes

REFERENCES

1. American Heart Association (AHA) — Pediatric Advanced Life Support (PALS) Guidelines 2020; with ILCOR focused updates. https://cpr.heart.org — Accessed August 2025.

2. Canadian Paediatric Society (CPS) — Position Statements and Practice Points. https://cps.ca — Accessed August 2025.

3. Canadian Pediatric Surveillance Program (CPSP) — Surveillance updates. https://www.cpsp.cps.ca — Accessed August 2025.

4. Public Health Agency of Canada — Canadian Immunization Guide. https://www.canada.ca — Accessed August 2025.

5. Centers for Disease Control and Prevention (CDC) — MIS-C guidance. https://www.cdc.gov — Accessed August 2025.

6. World Health Organization (WHO) — Pocket Book of Hospital Care for Children. https://www.who.int — Accessed August 2025.

7. NICE — Bronchiolitis in Children (NG9 or successor). https://www.nice.org.uk — Accessed August 2025.

8. Pediatric Emergency Care Applied Research Network (PECARN) — Clinical Decision Rules (Head Injury; Cervical Spine Injury). https://www.pecarn.org — Accessed August 2025.

9. American Academy of Pediatrics (AAP) — Hyperbilirubinemia guideline. https://www.aap.org — Accessed August 2025.

10. Canadian Thoracic Society — Asthma & Respiratory Guidelines. https://cts-sct.ca — Accessed August 2025.

Further Reading (Open Web)

1. PEMsource.org — Pediatric emergency algorithms (open web). Do not reproduce figures; cite only. https://pemsource.org — Accessed August 2025.